A Text Book Of

HUMAN ANATOMY AND PHYSIOLOGY - II

As Per PCI Regulations

FIRST YEAR B. PHARM.
Semester II

Dr. (Mrs.) Deepa S. Mandlik

M. Pharm, Ph.D. (Pharmacology)
Assistant Professor
Bharati Vidyapeeth's, Poona College of Pharmacy,
Erandwane
Pune - 411038, India

Prof. Satish K. Mandlik

M. Pharm (Quality Assurance)
Assistant Professor
Department of Pharmaceutics
STES's, Sinhgad College of Pharmacy
Vadgaon (Bk), Pune-411041, India

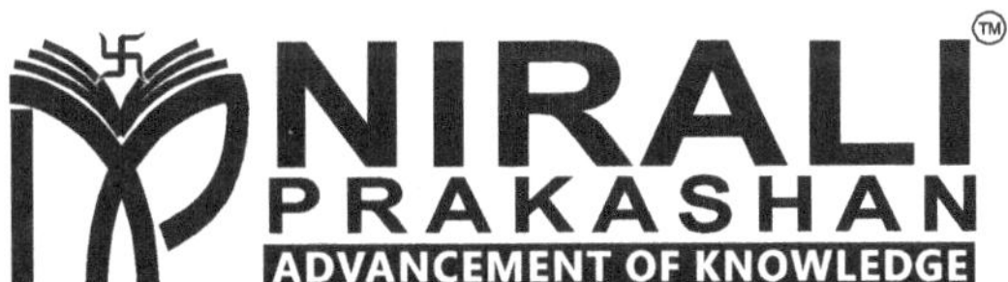

N3947

Human Anatomy and Physiology - II   ISBN 978-93-88897-99-0

Second Edition :   February 2020

© : **Authors**

Published By :
NIRALI PRAKASHAN
Abhyudaya Pragati, 1312, Shivaji Nagar,
Off J.M. Road, PUNE – 411005
Tel - (020) 25512336/37/39, Fax - (020) 25511379
Email : niralipune@pragationline.com

➢ DISTRIBUTION CENTRES

PUNE

Nirali Prakashan : 119, Budhwar Peth, Jogeshwari Mandir Lane, Pune 411002, Maharashtra
(For orders within Pune)   Tel : (020) 2445 2044, 66022708, Fax : (020) 2445 1538; Mobile : 9657703145
Email : niralilocal@pragationline.com

Nirali Prakashan : S. No. 28/27, Dhayari, Near Asian College Pune 411041
(For orders outside Pune)   Tel : (020) 24690204 Fax : (020) 24690316; Mobile : 9657703143
Email : bookorder@pragationline.com

MUMBAI

Nirali Prakashan : 385, S.V.P. Road, Rasdhara Co-op. Hsg. Society Ltd.,
Girgaum, Mumbai 400004, Maharashtra; Mobile : 9320129587
Tel : (022) 2385 6339 / 2386 9976, Fax : (022) 2386 9976
Email : niralimumbai@pragationline.com

➢ DISTRIBUTION BRANCHES

JALGAON

Nirali Prakashan : 34, V. V. Golani Market, Navi Peth, Jalgaon 425001, Maharashtra,
Tel : (0257) 222 0395, Mob : 94234 91860; Email : niralijalgaon@pragationline.com

KOLHAPUR

Nirali Prakashan : New Mahadvar Road, Kedar Plaza, 1st Floor Opp. IDBI Bank, Kolhapur 416 012
Maharashtra. Mob : 9850046155; Email : niralikolhapur@pragationline.com

NAGPUR

Nirali Prakashan : Above Maratha Mandir, Shop No. 3, First Floor,
Rani Jhanshi Square, Sitabuldi, Nagpur 440012, Maharashtra
Tel : (0712) 254 7129; Email : niralinagpur@pragationline.com

DELHI

Nirali Prakashan : 4593/15, Basement, Agarwal Lane, Ansari Road, Daryaganj
Near Times of India Building, New Delhi 110002 Mob : 08505972553
Email : niralidelhi@pragationline.com

BENGALURU

Nirali Prakashan : Maitri Ground Floor, Jaya Apartments, No. 99, 6th Cross, 6th Main,
Malleswaram, Bengaluru 560003, Karnataka; Mob : 9449043034
Email: niralibangalore@pragationline.com

Other Branches : Hyderabad, Chennai

niralipune@pragationline.com | www.pragationline.com
Also find us on www.facebook.com/niralibooks

Acknowledgement

We feel thankful to Hon'ble Late Dr. Patangrao Kadam (Founder President) and Hon'ble Dr. Vishwajeet Kadam (Chancellor), Bharati Vidyapeeth's Deemed University, Pune for their continuous encouragement and support for the publication of this book.

We are sincerely grateful to Dr. K. R. Mahadik, Principal and Dr. A. P. Pawar, Vice-Principal, Bharati Vidyapeeth's, Poona College of Pharmacy, Pune for their support, help and guidance.

We express sincere gratitude to Dr. K. S. Jain, K. K. Wagh College of Pharmacy, Nashik, Dr. (Mrs.). S. S. Patel, Institute of Pharmacy, Ahmadabad; Dr. R. V. Shete, R.D. College of Pharmacy, Bhor, Dr. N.S. Vyawahare, D. Y. Patil College of Pharmacy Pune for their continuous help, valuable guidance and advice.

We also express our gratitude to our all colleagues for their help and support during writing of this book.

We also express our special thanks to our parents, family members and our son Master Vignanshu Mandlik for their moral support.

We express our thanks to Prof. S. B. Gokhale, G. S. Redkar and staff members of Nirali Prakashan.

We are thankful to publisher Mr. Dineshbhai K. Furia, Mr. Jigneshbhai C. Furia, Mr. Malik Shaikh, Mrs. Roshan Shaikh and Mrs. Anjali Muley of Nirali Prakashan for their co-operation to publish this book.

Dr. Deepa S. Mandlik

Prof. Satish K. Mandlik

Preface

It gives us immense pleasure to introduce the book "**Textbook of Human Anatomy and Physiology**" for Semester - II.

Human anatomy gives knowledge regarding scientific study of morphology of the human body. Human physiology deals with functioning of body organs.

This book includes 08 chapters on human anatomy and physiology. The book is written in a simple and easy language along with schematics diagrams and tables. At the start of chapter learning objectives are mentioned and at the end of chapter short answer and long answer questions are given.

I hope that students will appreciate this book as each chapter is represented in notes format which will be beneficial for students from examination point of view.

We will be grateful to all the readers who finally judge the quality of this book and suggestions for the same will be highly appreciated and incorporated in the next edition.

Deepa S. Mandlik
Prof. Satish K. Mandlik

Syllabus

Unit I 10 Hours

Nervous System

Organization of Nervous System, Neuron, Neuroglia, Classification and Properties of Nerve Fibre, Electrophysiology, Action Potential, Nerve Impulse, Receptors, Synapse, Neurotransmitters.

Central Nervous System: Meninges, Ventricles of Brain and Cerebrospinal Fluid. Structure and Functions of Brain (Cerebrum, Brain stem, Cerebellum), Spinal Cord (Gross Structure, Functions of Afferent and Efferent Nerve Tracts, Reflex Activity).

Unit II 06 Hours

Digestive System

Anatomy of GI Tract with Special Reference to Anatomy and Functions of Stomach, (Acid Production in the Stomach, Regulation of Acid Production through Parasympathetic Nervous System, Pepsin Role in Protein Digestion) Small Intestine and Large Intestine, Anatomy and Functions of Salivary Glands, Pancreas and Liver, Movements of GIT, Digestion and Absorption of Nutrients and Disorders of GIT.

Energetics

Formation and role of ATP, Creatinine Phosphate and BMR.

Unit III 10 Hours

Respiratory System

Anatomy of Respiratory System with Special Reference to Anatomy of Lungs, Mechanism of Respiration, Regulation of Respiration. Lung Volumes and Capacities Transport of Respiratory Gases, Artificial Respiration, and Resuscitation Methods.

Urinary System

Anatomy of Urinary Tract with Special Reference to Anatomy of Kidney and Nephrons, Functions of Kidney and Urinary Tract, Physiology of Urine Formation, Micturition Reflex and Role of Kidneys in Acid Base Balance, Role of RAS in Kidney and Disorders of kidney.

Unit IV 10 Hours

Endocrine System

Classification of Hormones, Mechanism of Hormone Action, Structure and Functions of Pituitary Gland, Thyroid Gland, Parathyroid Gland, Adrenal Gland, Pancreas, Pineal Gland, Thymus and their Disorders.

Unit V 09 Hours

Reproductive System

Anatomy of Male and Female Reproductive System, Functions of Male and Female Reproductive System, Sex Hormones, Physiology of Menstruation, Fertilization, Spermatogenesis, Oogenesis, Pregnancy and Parturition.

Introduction to Genetics

Chromosomes, Genes and DNA, Protein Synthesis, Genetic Pattern of Inheritance.

***

Contents

UNIT III

3. Energetics   3.1 - 3.8

UNIT III

4. Respiratory System   4.1 - 4.24

***

UNIT I

Chapter 1 ...

NERVOUS SYSTEM

♦ LEARNING OBJECTIVES ♦

- ❖ To classify the nervous system.
- ❖ To describe the three basic functions of the nervous system.
- ❖ To describe the structure of neuron.
- ❖ To explain the formation and circulation of cerebrospinal fluid.
- ❖ To describe the structure and function of cerebrum.
- ❖ To describe the structure and function of basal ganglia.
- ❖ To describe the structures and functions of limbic system.
- ❖ To describe the locations and functions of the sensory, association, and motor areas of the cerebral cortex.
- ❖ To describe the structures and functions of the brain stem.
- ❖ To describe the structure and functions of the cerebellum.
- ❖ To describe the components and functions of the diencephalon.
- ❖ To identify the cranial nerves by name, number, and type and give the functions of each nerve.
- ❖ To compare the sympathetic and parasympathetic divisions of the autonomic nervous system.
- ❖ To describe the protective covering, internal and external anatomy of spinal cord.
- ❖ To describe the functional components of a reflex arc.

1.1 INTRODUCTION

The nervous system coordinates the voluntary and involuntary movements of the human body and transmits signals between different body parts. The nervous system detects and responds to changes inside and outside the body. Together with the endocrine system, it controls important aspects of body function and maintains homeostasis. The nervous system regulates various activities of the body by responding rapidly using nerve impulses (action potentials) whereas, the endocrine system responds more slowly by releasing different hormones from glands.

The branch of medical science that deals with the structure, functions and diseases of the nervous system is called Neurology.

1.2 DIVISIONS OF THE NERVOUS SYSTEM

- The two principle divisions of the nervous system are the Central Nervous System (CNS) and Peripheral Nervous System (PNS).

(1.1)

- The CNS consists of brain and spinal cord, which together integrate and correlate many different kinds of incoming sensory information.
- The CNS is also the source of thoughts, emotions and memories.
- The components of Peripheral Nervous System (PNS) are subdivided into a Somatic Nervous System (SNS) and Autonomic Nervous System (ANS).
- The SNS is voluntary.
- The SNS consist of sensory neurons and motor neurons.
  - ✓ **Sensory neurons:** They convey information from somatic receptors in the head, body wall, limbs and from receptors of special senses of vision, hearing, taste and smell to the CNS.
  - ✓ **Motor neurons:** They conduct impulses from the CNS to skeletal muscles.
- The ANS is involuntary.
- The ANS consists of sympathetic and parasympathetic division.
  - ✓ **Sensory neurons:** They convey information from autonomic sensory receptors, located primarily in visceral organs such as stomach and lungs to the CNS.
  - ✓ **Motor neurons:** They conduct nerve impulses from the CNS to smooth muscles, cardiac muscles and glands.

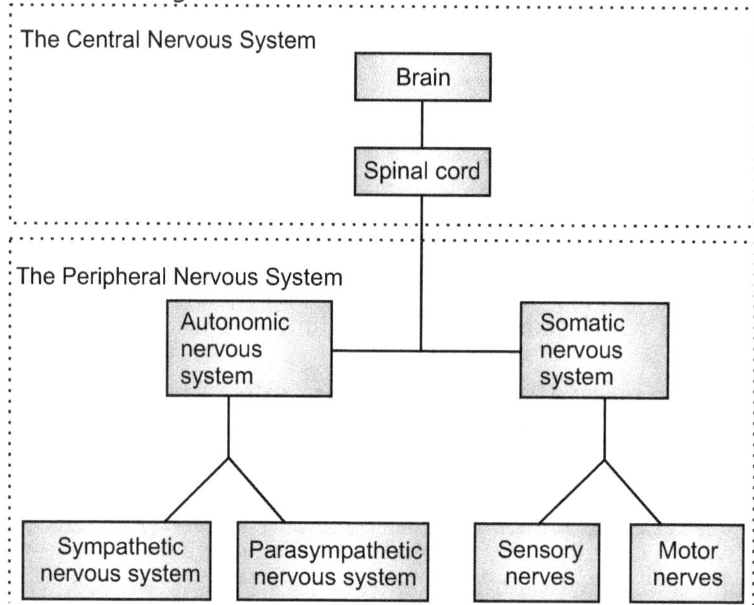

Fig. 1.1: Organization of the nervous system

Functions

The functions of nervous system can be grouped into 3 parts.

Sensory function

- Sensory receptors detect internal stimuli such as increase in blood acidity and external stimuli such as rain drop falling on the arm.
- This sensory information is then carried to the brain and spinal cord through cranial and spinal nerves.

Integrative function

- The nervous system integrates and processes sensory information by analyzing and making decisions of appropriate responses.
- The neurons involved in these processes are called as interneurons.

Motor function

- The motor function involves responding to integration decision by activating effectors (muscle or glands) through cranial or spinal nerves.
- The neurons which serve these functions are called as motor or afferent neuron.
- Stimulation of the effector organs causes muscles to contract and secretion of hormones from glands.

1.3 HISTOLOGY OF NEURON

- Neuron is the fundamental unit of the nervous system.
- Nervous system consists of two types of cells.
  - ✓ Neurons
  - ✓ Neuroglia
- Neurons perform the function of sensing, thinking, remembering, controlling muscle activity and regulating glandular secretions.
- Neuroglia support, nourish and protect the neurons and maintain homeostasis in the interstitial fluid that bathes the neurons.

1.3.1 Neuron

Neuron is composed of three parts:

- ✓ Cell body
- ✓ Dendrites
- ✓ Axon

Cell body

- It contains a nucleus surrounded by a cytoplasm that includes various organelles such as lysosomes, mitochondria and golgi complex.
- Two kinds of processes emerge from the cell body of neuron i.e. multiple dendrites and a single axon.

Dendrites

- These are short, tapering and highly branched.
- Each nerve cell contains many dendrites.
- These are input portion of a neuron and receive signals from sense organs or from the axons of the other neurons.
- These signals are converted into electrical impulses and transmitted to the cell body.

Axon

- It is a long, thin, cylindrical projection that joins the cell body.
- The cone shaped elevation is called the axon hillock.
- It is the major output portion of the neuron that conducts nerve impulses away from the cell body.
- The first part of the axon is initial segment.
- An axon contains mitochondria, microtubules and neurofibrils.

- The cytoplasm of axon called as axoplasm is surrounded by a plasma membrane known as axolemma.
- Along the length of an axon, many branches are present called as axon collaterals.
- The axon and its collateral end by dividing into many fine processes called as axon terminals.
- The site of communication between two neurons or between a neuron and an effector cell is called as synapse.
- The tip of axon terminals swells into bulb shaped structures called as synaptic bulb ends.
- Synaptic end bulbs contain many tiny membrane enclosed sacs called as synaptic vesicles that store a chemical neurotransmitter.
- When neurotransmitter molecules are released from synaptic vesicles they excite or inhibit other neurons, muscle fibres or gland cell.

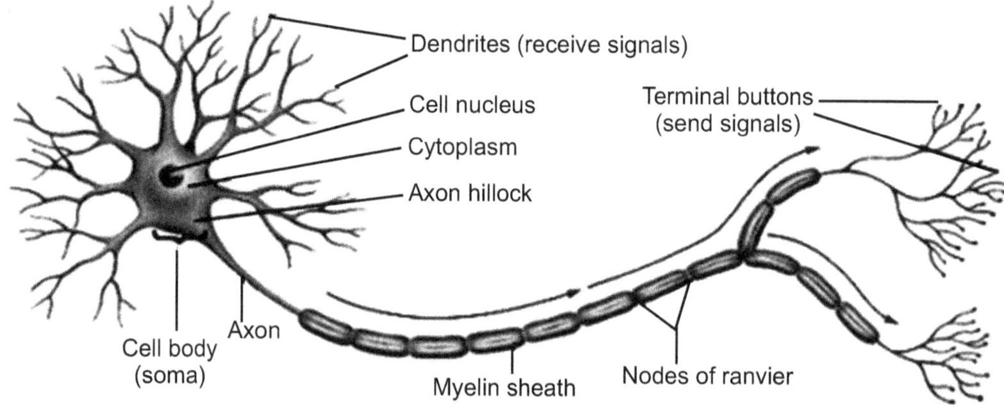

Fig. 1.2: Neuron

1.3.2 Types of Neurons

- Neurons are classified according to the number of processes extending from the cell body.

Multipolar neuron

- They have several dendrites and one axon
- E.g. Brain and spinal cord

Bipolar neuron

- They have one main dendrite and one axon
- E.g. Retina of eye, inner ear and olfactory area of the brain

Unipolar neuron

- These are sensory neurons that begin in the embryo as bipolar neurons.
- During development, the axon and dendrites fuse into a single process that divides into two branches a short distance from the cell body.

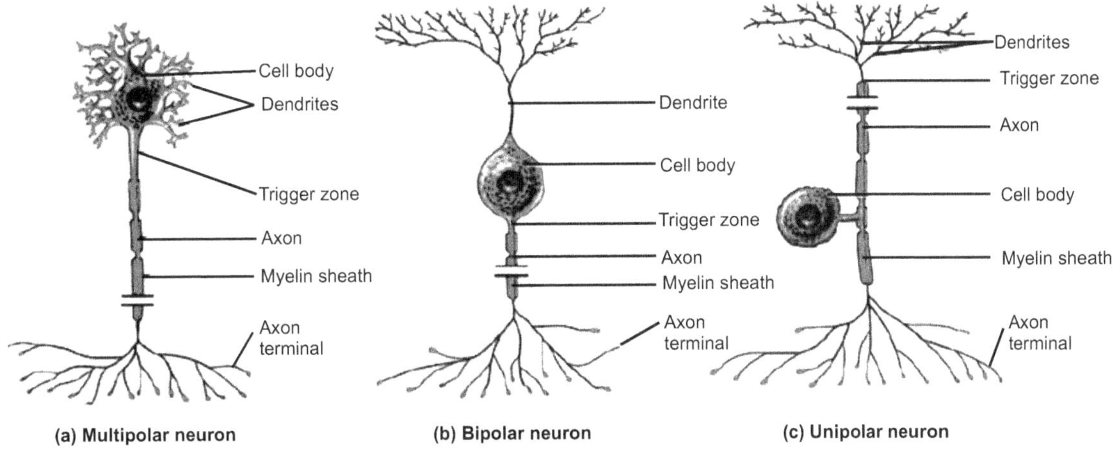

Fig. 1.3: Types of neurons

1.3.3 Neuroglia (Glia)

- It constitute about half the volume of the CNS. These are smaller than neurons.
- They do not generate action potential and they can multiply and divide in the mature nervous system.

Types of Neuroglia

✓ Astrocytes
✓ Oligodendrocytes
✓ Microglia
✓ Ependymal cells
✓ Schwann cells
✓ Satellite cells

Astrocytes

- These are star shaped cells with many processes.
- They maintain appropriate environment for generation of nerve impulses, provide nutrients to neurons, take up excess neurotransmitter, help form the blood brain barrier.

Oligodendrocytes

- These are smaller than astrocytes, with fewer processes, round or oval body.
- They form supporting network around CNS neurons; produce myelin sheath around several adjacent axons of CNS neurons.

Microglia

- These are small cells with few processes, derived from mesodermal cells that also give rise to monocytes and macrophages.
- They protect CNS cells from disease by engulfing invading microbes to areas of injured nerve tissue where they clear away debris of dead cells.

Ependymal cells

- These are arranged in a single layer, ranges in shape from cuboidal to columnar, many are ciliated.

- It lines the ventricles of the brain and central canal of the spinal cord, forms cerebrospinal fluid and assists in its circulation.

Schwann cells

- These are flattened cells that encircle PNS axons.
- Each cell surrounds multiple unmyelinated axons with a single layer of its plasma membrane or produces part of myelin sheath around a single axon of a PNS neuron.
- They participate in regeneration of PNS axons.

Satellite cells

- These are flattened cells arranged around the cell bodies of neurons in ganglia.
- They support neurons in PNS ganglia.

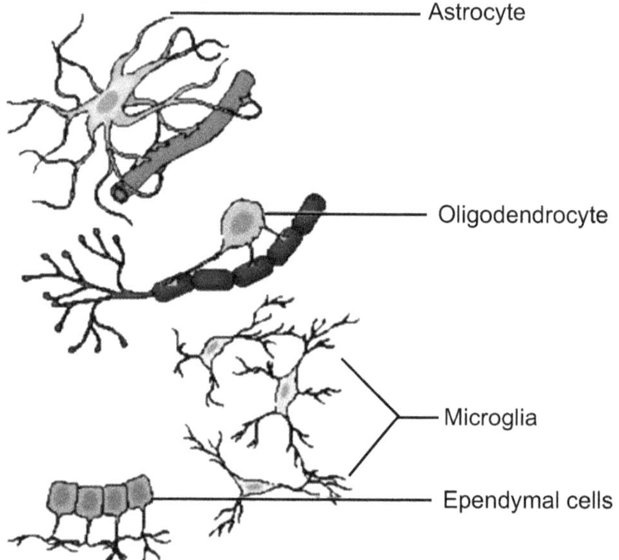

Fig. 1.4: Types of Neuroglia

1.4 CLASSIFICATION OF NERVE FIBERS

- Axons are divided into three types depending on the size and speed of conduction.

1. A fibers:

- These are myelinated and largest-diameter axons (5–20 μm).
- These fibers are the thickest and fastest conducting.
- A fibers have an absolute refractory period and conduct nerve impulses at speeds of 12 to 130 m/sec.
- Examples of type A fibers are skeleton-motor fibers, fusi-motor fibers and afferent fibers to skin.

2. B fibers:

- These fibers are medium in size (2–3 μm), i.e. they are smaller than type A fibers but larger than type C.
- They are myelinated.
- Their speed of conduction is 3-15 m/sec, which shows that they are slower than type A fibers.

- B fibers conduct sensory nerve impulses from the viscera to the brain and spinal cord.
- They consist of axons of the autonomic motor neurons that extend from the brain and spinal cord to the ANS.

3. C fibers:

- These fibers are smallest in diameter (0.5–1.5 μm) and thinnest.
- They are non-myelinated.
- Their speed of conduction is 0.5-4 m/sec, which shows that they have the slowest conduction speed.
- These unmyelinated axons conduct sensory impulses for pain, touch, pressure, heat, and cold from the skin, and pain impulses from the viscera.
- Autonomic motor fibers that extend from autonomic ganglia to stimulate the heart, smooth muscle, and glands are C fibers.

1.5 PROPERTIES OF NERVE FIBERS

Excitability:

- When a stimulus is applied, the nerve fiber demonstrates a change in its electrical activity from its resting state.

Conductivity:

- It is the ability of the nerve fiber to transmit impulses all along the whole length of axon without any change in the amplitude of the action potential. This type of conduction is termed as decrementless conduction.

Refractory period:

- It is the duration after an effective stimulus, when a second stimulus is applied, there will be no response for the second stimulus.
- Relative refractory period is the duration after an effective stimulus, when a second stimulus, which is slightly above threshold, is applied there will be response for the second stimulus as well.

All or none law:

- It states that, when the tissue is stimulated with threshold or more than threshold strength, the amplitude of response will remain the same but for a stimulus of less than threshold strength; there will not be any response.

1.6 GENERATION OF ACTION POTENTIAL

Resting membrane potential

- There is normally a charge difference across the plasma membrane of a neuron.
- The value of resting membrane potential is −70 mV.
- The outside of the membrane has a positive charge and inside has a negative charge.
- Resting potential results from differences between sodium and potassium positively charged ions and negatively charged ions in the cytoplasm.

- Sodium ions are more concentrated outside the membrane, while potassium ions are more concentrated inside the membrane.
- This imbalance is maintained by the active transport of ions across the membrane known as the sodium potassium pump.
- The resting potential is usually about -70 mv.

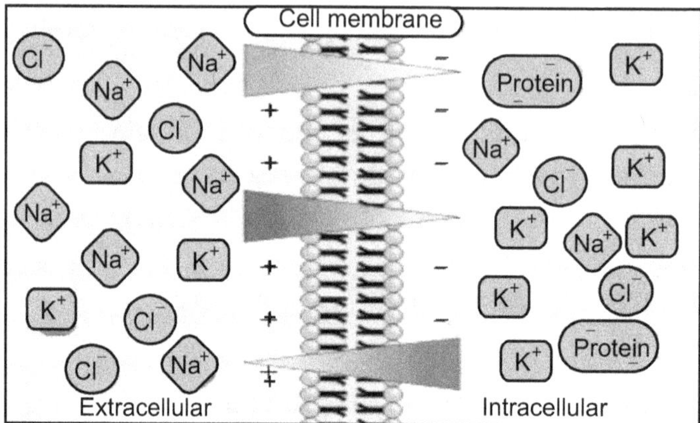

Fig. 1.5: Concentration of sodium and potassium ions across the cell membrane

Action Potential (AP)

- It is a momentary change in the membrane potential caused by a transient change in the membrane's permeability to sodium and potassium ions.
- When a neuron receives signals, an abrupt, temporary reversal in the polarity is generated (an action potential).
- The inside of membrane becomes more positive.
- Due to change in voltage, the voltage-gated channels in the membrane get opens.
- As a result of ion flow through these channels, the inside of a neuron briefly becomes more positive than outside.
- AP has three main phases:
    - **Depolarizing phase:** The negative membrane potential becomes less negative, reaches zero, and then becomes positive.
    - **Repolarizing phase:** The membrane potential is restored to the resting state of -70 mV.
    - **After-hyperpolarizing phase:** The membrane potential temporarily becomes more negative than the resting level.

Types of voltage-gated channels

- Two types of voltage gated channels open and close during action potential.
- The channels are present mainly in the axon plasma membrane and axon terminals.
- **Voltage-gated Na⁺ channels:** The voltage-gated Na⁺ channels open, allowing Na⁺ ions to rush into the cell, which causes the depolarizing phase.

- **Voltage-gated K+ channels:** Then voltage-gated K^+ channels open, allowing K^+ to flow out, which produces the repolarizing phase.

Phases of action potential

- There are five important phase of action potential.
  - ✓ Threshold Phase
  - ✓ Depolarizing Phase
  - ✓ Repolarizing Phase
  - ✓ After-hyperpolarizing Phase
  - ✓ Refractory period

Threshold Phase

- The threshold potential is the critical level to which the membrane potential must be depolarized in order to initiate an action potential.
- The value of threshold potential is -55 mV.
- When a stimulus depolarizes the membrane to threshold, an AP is generated.
- The action potential arises then propagates along the axon to the axon terminals.
- The axon plasma membrane and axon terminals of the neuron have voltage-gated Na^+ and K^+ channels.
- Threshold stimulus, is a stimulus strong enough to depolarize the membrane to threshold.
- Suprathreshold stimulus, is a stimulus strong enough to depolarize the membrane above the threshold.

Depolarizing Phase

- When a depolarizing graded potential or some other stimulus causes the axon membrane to depolarize to threshold, voltage-gated Na^+ channels open rapidly.
- Both the electrical and chemical gradients favour inward movement of Na^+ ions and the resulting inflow of Na^+ ions causes the depolarizing phase of the action potential.
- The inflow of Na^+ ions changes the membrane potential from -55 mV to -30 mV.
- At the peak of the action potential, the inside of the membrane is 30 mV more positive than the outside.
- Each voltage gated Na^+ channel has two separate gates, an activation gate and an inactivation gate.
- In the resting state of a voltage-gated Na^+ channel, the inactivation gate is open, but the activation gate is closed.
- As a result, Na^+ ions cannot move into the cell through these channels.
- At threshold, the voltage-gated Na^+ channels are activated.
- In the activated state of a voltage-gated Na^+ channel, both the activation and inactivation gates in the channel are open and Na^+ inflow begins.

- As more channels open, Na^+ inflow increases, the membrane depolarizes further and more Na^+ channels get open.

Repolarizing Phase

- After a short period, the activation gates of voltage gated Na^+ channels open, the inactivation gates close.
- The voltage-gated Na^+ channel is in an inactivated state.
- In addition to opening voltage-gated Na^+ channels, a threshold level depolarization also opens voltage-gated K^+ channels.
- Because the voltage-gated K^+ channels open more slowly, their opening occurs at about the same time the voltage-gated Na^+ channels are closing.
- The slower opening of voltage-gated K^+ channels and the closing of previously open voltage-gated Na^+ channels produce the repolarizing phase of the action potential.
- As the Na^+ channels are inactivated, Na^+ ions inflow slows. At the same time, the K^+ channels are opening, accelerating K^+ ions outflow.
- Slowing of Na^+ ions inflow and acceleration of K^+ ions outflow causes the membrane potential to change from -30 mV to -70 mV.
- Repolarization also allows inactivated Na^+ channels to revert to the resting state.

After-hyperpolarizing Phase

- When the voltage-gated K^+ channels are open, outflow of K^+ ions may be large enough to cause an after-hyperpolarizing phase of the action potential.
- During this phase, the voltage-gated K^+ channels remain open and the membrane potential becomes even more negative (about -90 mV).
- As the voltage-gated K^+ channels closes, the membrane potential returns to the resting level of -70 mV.

Refractory Period

- The period of time after an action potential begins during which an excitable cell cannot generate another action potential in response to a normal threshold stimulus is called the refractory period.
- Refractory period, which returns potassium ions to inside of the cell and sodium ions to outside of the cell.
- The sodium-potassium pump goes back to work, moving Na^+ ions to the outside of the cell and K^+ ions to the inside, returning the neuron to its normal polarized state.
- Two types of refractory periods are there.
- **Absolute refractory period (ARP):** The period from the initiation of the action potential to immediately after the peak is referred as the absolute refractory period (ARP).
- **Relative refractory period (RRP):** The period during which a stronger than normal stimulus is needed in order to elicit an action potential is referred as the relative refractory period (RRP).

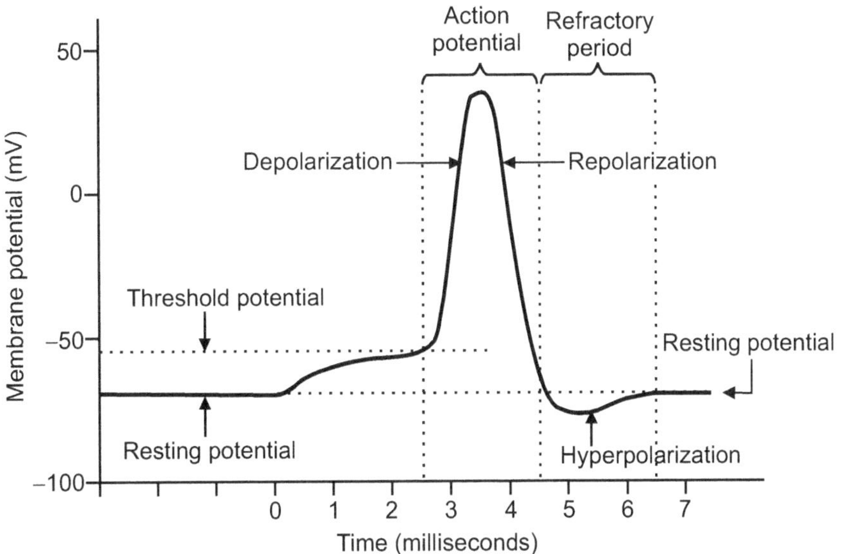

Fig. 1.6: Events in Action potential

1.7 NEUROTRANSMITTERS (NT's)

- Neurotransmitters are synthesized in the nerve endings.
- Enzymes and precursor molecules are required for NT synthesis.
- Once synthesized, the NT is protected from enzymatic degradation by storage in vesicle.
- A nerve action potential causes release of NT into the synaptic space or the neuro-effector junction.
- The liberated NT then attaches to the effector cell membrane, resulting in depolarization and generation of action potential.
- Two basic NT's are involved in automous nervous system are acetylcholine and nor-epinephrine.

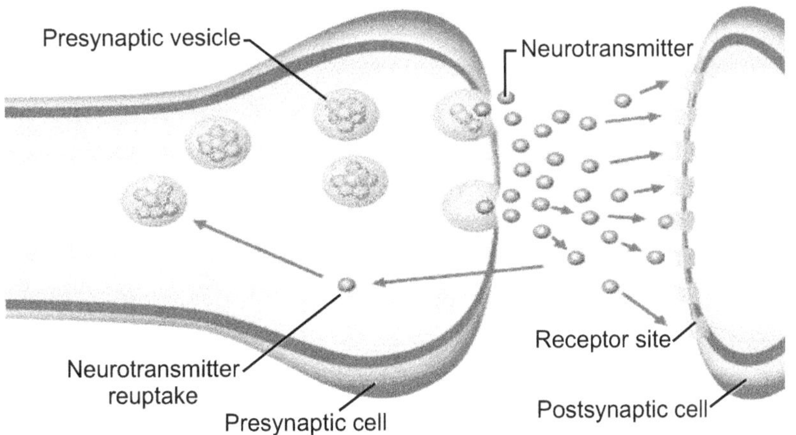

Fig. 1.7: Storage and release of neurotransmitter

Types of neurotransmitters are:

✓ Small molecules NTs
✓ Neuropeptides

Small molecules NTs

- These are rapidly acting small molecule neurotransmitters that produce responses.
  - ✓ Acetylcholine
  - ✓ Norepinephrine
  - ✓ Epinephrine
  - ✓ Dopamine
  - ✓ Serotonin

Different amino acids

- ✓ Glycine
- ✓ Gamma-amino-butyric acid (GABA)
- ✓ Aspartate
- ✓ Glutamate

Neuropeptides

- These are slowly acting NT's having prolonged effects.
- These hormones are released from the hypothalamus E.g. Thyroid stimulating Phormone, Somatostatin, etc.
  - ✓ **Pituitary peptides:** E.g. Adrenocorticotropin hormone, Vasopressin, Oxytocin, etc.
  - ✓ **Peptides acting on gut and brain:** E.g. Substance P, Insulin, Glucagon, Enkephalin, etc.
  - ✓ **Neuropeptides from other tissues:** E.g. Bradykinin, Angiotensin-II, etc.

Acetylcholine (Ach)

- It is a NT released by many peripheral nervous system neurons and by some central nervous system neurons.
- It is an excitatory NT at neuromuscular junction, where it acts directly to open ligand-gated cation channels.
- It is also acts as inhibitory NT at other synapses where its effect on ion channel is indirect via receptors that link to G protein.
- The enzyme acetyl cholinesterase (AchE) inactivates Ach by splitting it into acetate and choline.

Biogenic amines

- Certain amino acids are modified and decarboxylated to produce biogenic amines.
- Norepinephrine plays an important role in awakening from deep sleep, dreaming and regulating mood.
- Smaller number of neurons in the brain use epinephrine as a NT.
- Brain neurons containing the NT dopamine are active during emotional and pleasurable responses.
- Dopamine releasing neurons also helps to regulate the skeletal muscle tone.
- Schizophrenia occurs due to the accumulation of excess dopamine.
- Muscular stiffness occurs due to the degeneration of neurons that release dopamine in Parkinson's disease.
- Serotonin plays an important role in sensory perception, temperature regulation, control of mood, appetite and induction of sleep.

1.8 NEUROTRANSMITTER RECEPTORS

- It is also known as a neuroreceptor is a membrane receptor protein that is activated by a neurotransmitter.
- Chemicals on the outside of cell, such as a neurotransmitter, can bump on to the cell's membrane.
- If a neurotransmitter bumps into its corresponding receptor, they will bind and can trigger other events to occur inside the cell.
- Therefore, a membrane receptor is part of the molecular machinery that allows cells to communicate with one another.
- A neurotransmitter receptor is a class of receptors that specifically binds with neurotransmitters as opposed to other molecules.
- Each type of neurotransmitter receptor has one or more neurotransmitter binding sites where its specific neurotransmitter binds.
- When a neurotransmitter binds to the correct neurotransmitter receptor, an ion channel opens and a postsynaptic potential forms in the membrane of the postsynaptic cell.
- Neurotransmitter receptors are classified as either ionotropic or metabotropic receptors depending on the basis of neurotransmitter binding site and the ion channel.

Ionotropic Receptors

- It is a type of ligand-gated channel.
- It is a type of neurotransmitter receptor that contains a neurotransmitter binding site and the ion channel.
- The neurotransmitter binding site and the ion channel are components of the same protein.
- In absence of neurotransmitter (the ligand), the ion channel component of the ionotropic receptor is closed.
- When the exact neurotransmitter binds to the ionotropic receptor, the ion channel get opens, and an excitatory or inhibitory postsynaptic potential occurs in the postsynaptic cell.
- Many excitatory neurotransmitters bind to ionotropic receptors that contain cation channels such as Na^+, K^+ and Ca^{2+}.
- When cation channels gets open, they allow passage of the three most abundant cations through the postsynaptic cell membrane causes excitatory postsynaptic potential.
- But Na^+ ion inflow is greater than either Ca^{2+} ion inflow or K^+ ion outflow and the inside of the cell becomes less negative (depolarized).
- Many inhibitory neurotransmitters bind to ionotropic receptors that contain chloride channels such as Cl^-.
- When Cl^- channels open, a larger number of chloride ions diffuse inward.
- The inward flow of Cl^- ions causes the inside of postsynaptic cell to become more negative (hyperpolarized) and causes inhibitory postsynaptic potential.

Metabotropic Receptors

- It is a type of neurotransmitter receptor that contains a neurotransmitter binding site, but lacking an ion channel.
- It is coupled to a separate ion channel by a membrane protein called as G protein.
- When a neurotransmitter binds to a metabotropic receptor, the G protein either directly opens or closes the ion channel or it may act indirectly by activating a second messenger in the cytosol, which in turn opens or closes the ion channel.
- Thus, a metabotropic receptor is different from an ionotropic receptor in that the neurotransmitter binding site and the ion channel are modules of different proteins.
- Some inhibitory neurotransmitters bind to metabotropic receptors that are linked to K^+ channels.
- When K^+ channels open, a larger number of K^+ ions diffuses outside the membrane that results into generation of inhibitory postsynaptic potential.
- The outward flow of K^+ ions causes the inside of the postsynaptic cell to become more negative (hyperpolarized).

1.9 SYNAPSES

- It is a small gap at the end of a neuron where communication occurs between two neurons or between a neuron and an effector cell.
- Presynaptic neurons refer to a nerve cell that carries nerve impulses towards a synapse.
- Postsynaptic neurons that carries a nerve impulse away from a synapse or an effector cell that responds to the impulse at the synapse.

Parts of the Synapse

- These are composed of 3 main parts:
  - ✓ The presynaptic ending that contains neurotransmitters.
  - ✓ The synaptic cleft between the two nerve cells.
  - ✓ The postsynaptic ending that contains receptor sites.
- An electrical impulse travels along the length of axon and then causes the release of tiny vesicles containing neurotransmitters.
- These vesicles will then bind to the membrane of the presynaptic cell, releasing the neurotransmitters into the synapse.
- These chemical messengers cross the synaptic cleft and connect with receptor sites in the next nerve cell, triggering an electrical impulse known as an action potential.

Types of Synapses

- **Chemical Synapse**
  - The plasma membranes of presynaptic and postsynaptic neurons in a chemical synapse are separated by the synaptic cleft (a space of 20–50 nm) that is filled with interstitial fluid.

- As the nerve impulse enters, the presynaptic neuron releases a neurotransmitter in the synaptic cleft and binds to receptors in the plasma membrane of the postsynaptic neuron.

- The postsynaptic neuron receives the chemical signal and produces a postsynaptic potential called as graded potential.

- Thus, the presynaptic neuron converts an electrical signal (nerve impulse) into a chemical signal (released neurotransmitter).

- The postsynaptic neuron receives the chemical signal and in turn generates an electrical signal (postsynaptic potential).

- A typical chemical synapse transmits a signal as follows;

- A nerve impulse reaches at a synaptic end bulb of a presynaptic axon.

- The depolarizing phase of the nerve impulse opens voltage gated Ca^{2+} channels, present in the membrane of synaptic end bulbs so; there will be inflow of Ca^{2+} ions through the opened channels.

- Due to increase in the concentration of Ca^{2+} ions inside the presynaptic neuron triggers the exocytosis of synaptic vesicles.

- As vesicle membranes merge with the plasma membrane, neurotransmitter molecules within the vesicles are released into the synaptic cleft.

- Each synaptic vesicle contains several thousand molecules of neurotransmitter.

- The neurotransmitter molecules diffuse across the synaptic cleft and bind to neurotransmitter receptors in the postsynaptic neuron's plasma membrane.

- Binding of neurotransmitter molecules to the receptors on ligand-gated channels opens the channels and allows particular ions to flow across the membrane.

- Due to inflow of ions through the opened channels, there is change in the voltage across the membrane.

- This change in membrane voltage is called as postsynaptic potential.

- Depending on the type of ions enters the channel; the postsynaptic potential may be a depolarization or a hyperpolarization.

- For example, opening of Na^+ channels allows inflow of Na^+, which causes depolarization whereas; opening of Cl^- or K^+ channels causes hyperpolarization.

- When a depolarizing postsynaptic potential reaches threshold, it triggers an event of action potential in the axon of the postsynaptic neuron.

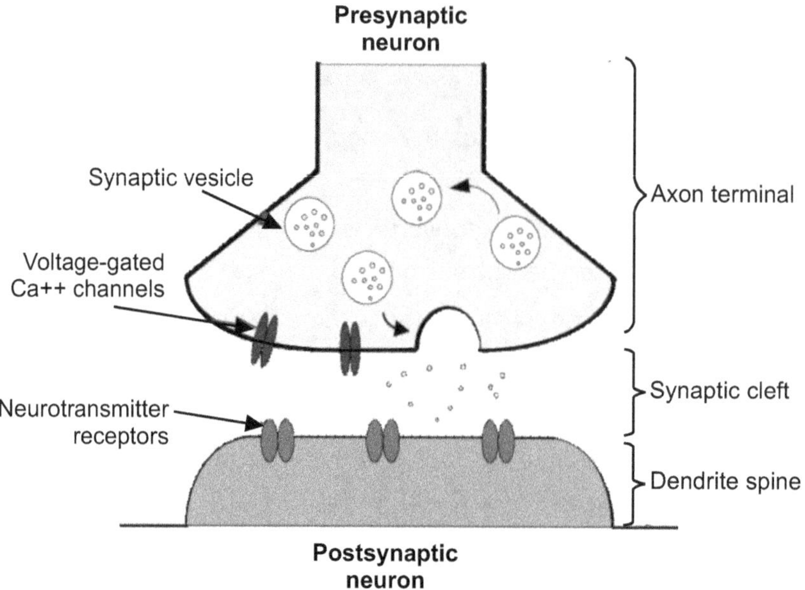

Fig. 1.8: Signal transmission at chemical synapse

Electrical Synapse

- In electrical synapse, two neurons are connected by specialized channels known as gap junctions.

- Electrical synapses allow electrical signals to travel quickly from the presynaptic cell to the postsynaptic cell, rapidly speeding up the transfer of signals.

- The gap between electrical synapses is much smaller than that of a chemical synapse.

- The special protein channels that connect the two cells make it possible for the positive current from the presynaptic neuron to flow directly into the postsynaptic cell.

- Electrical synapses transfer signals much faster than chemical synapses. Whereas; chemical synapses can be excitatory or inhibitory in nature, electrical synapses are excitatory only.

1.10 MENINGES OF BRAIN

- The cranium is the bony covering that protects the brain.
- The meninges lie between the brain and the spinal cord.
- They consist of three layers of tissue namely - dura mater, arachnoid mater and pia mater.
- The outermost layer is called the dura mater. It lines the inside of the skull and forms folds or compartments.
- The two special folds of the dura mater are called the falx and the tentorium.
- The falx separates the right and left half of the brain and the tentorium separates the upper and lower parts of the brain.

- The second layer of the meninges is the arachnoid mater. It covers the entire brain.
- The space between the dura and the arachnoid membranes is called the subdural space.
- The innermost layer of meninges is called the pia mater. It has many blood vessels that reach deep into surface of the brain.
- The space that separates the arachnoid and the pia mater is called the subarachnoid space. The extensions of the dura mater separate parts of the brain.
  - ✓ **Falx cerebri:** It separates the two hemispheres of the cerebrum.
  - ✓ **Falx cerebelli:** It separates the two hemispheres of the cerebellum.
  - ✓ **Tentorium cerebelli:** It separates the cerebrum from the cerebellum.

1.11 CEREBROSPINAL FLUID (CSF)

- Cerebrospinal fluid is present in the ventricles of brain, in cisterns around the brain and in the sub-arachnoid space around both the brain and the spinal cord.
- It is a clear, colourless liquid that protects the brain and spinal cord against chemical and physical injuries.
- It carries oxygen, glucose and other necessary chemicals from the blood to neurons and neuroglia.
- Approximately 500 ml of CSF is formed every day.
- The total volume of CSF is 80 to 150 ml in an adult.
- CSF contains glucose, proteins, lactic acid, urea, cations (Na^+, K^+, Ca^+, Mg^+) and anions (Cl^- and HCO_3^-).
- It also contains some white blood cells.

Functions
- It protects the delicate structure of the brain and the spinal cord.
- It acts as a shock absorber providing cushioning to the brain and the spinal cord.
- It maintains uniform pressure around these delicate structures.
- It provides chemical protection to the brain and the spinal cord.
- CSF is a medium for exchange of nutrients and waste products between the blood and the nervous tissue.

1.12 BRAIN

- It is one of the most complex organ of the human body.
- The brain controls thoughts, memory, speech, limb movements and the function of many organs within the body.
- It also determines how people respond to external stimulus and environment by regulating heart and breathing rates.
- It is an organised structure, divided into many components that serve specific and important functions.
- It consists of four major parts:
  - ✓ Cerebrum
  - ✓ Diencephalon
  - ✓ Cerebellum
  - ✓ Brain Stem

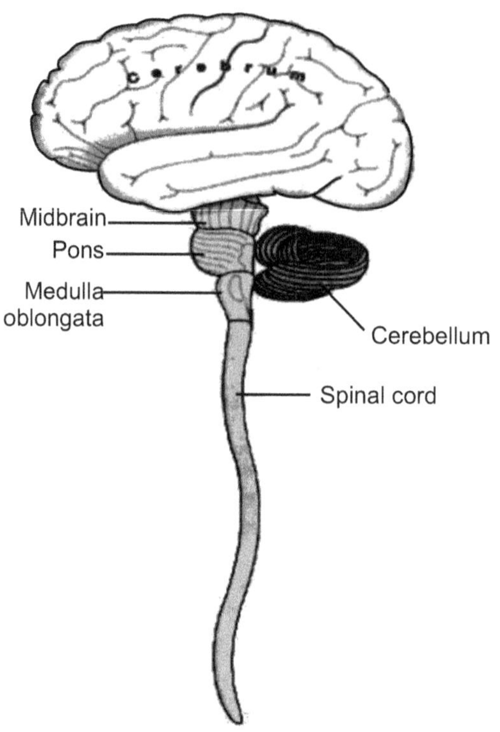

Fig. 1.9: Components of the nervous system

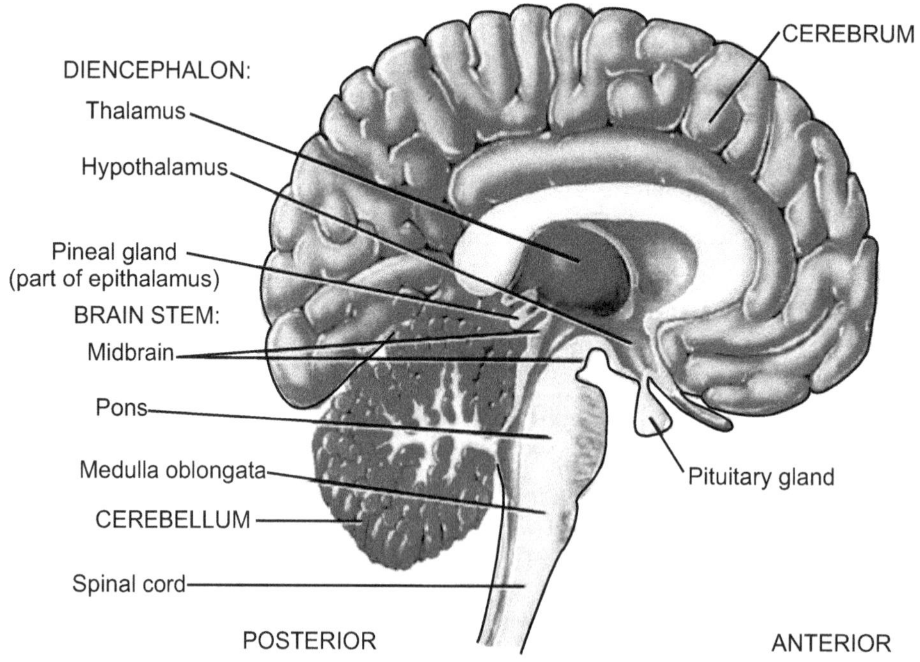

Fig. 1.10: Brain

1.13 CEREBRUM

- It is supported on the diencephalon and brain stem.
- It is the largest part of the brain.
- It is the seat of intelligence.
- It provides us with the ability to read, write and speak, to make calculations and compose music, to remember the past, plan for the future and imagine things that have never existed before.
- The right and left halves of the cerebrum is called as cerebral hemispheres.
- The superficial layer of the cerebrum is gray mater.
- This 2 - 4 mm thick gray superficial area contains billons of neurons.
- Below the gray mater is the white mater.
- The cerebrum shows folds of gray mater on the surface; these folds are called as *gyri*.
- If the grooves between folds are deep they are called *fissures* and if shallower they are called as sulci.
- The most prominent fissure, the longitudinal fissure, separates the cerebrum into right and left halves called as cerebral hemispheres.
- The hemispheres are connected internally by the corpus callosum a broad band of white mater.

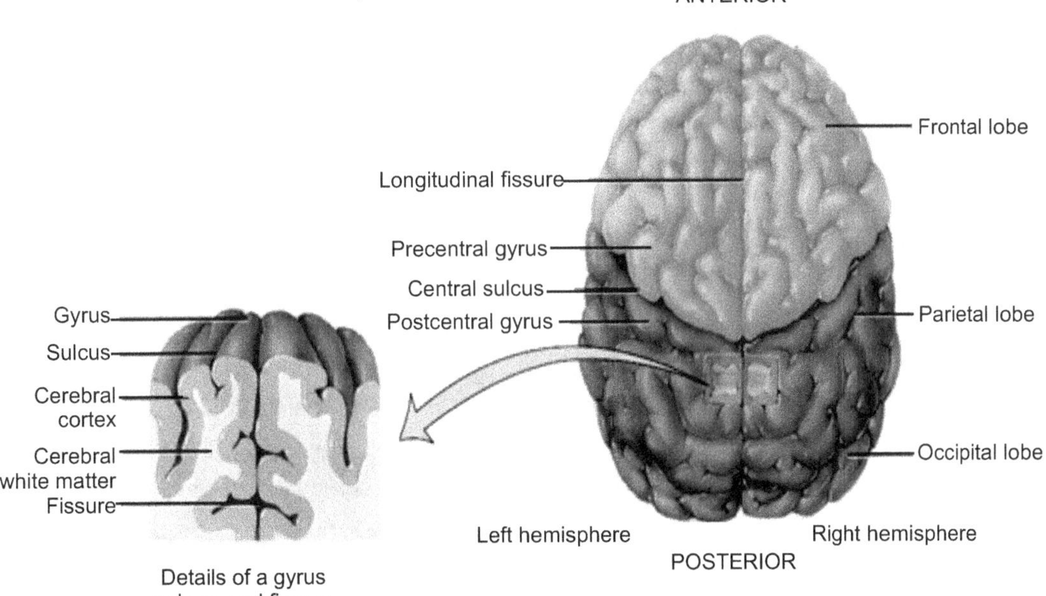

Fig. 1.11: Cerebral hemispheres and folds of cerebrum

1.13.1 Lobes and Functional Areas of Cerebrum

- Each cerebral hemisphere is further subdivided into four lobes.
- ✓ Frontal lobe
- ✓ Parietal lobe
- ✓ Temporal lobe
- ✓ Occipital lobe

- A major gyrus, the precentral gyrus located immediately anterior to the central sulcus separates the frontal lobe from the parietal lobe.
- The lateral cerebral sulcus separates the frontal lobe from the temporal lobe.
- The parieto-occipital sulcus separates the parietal lobe from the occipital lobe.
- A fifth part of the cerebrum, the insula cannot be seen at the surface of the brain because it lies within the lateral cerebral sulcus, deep to the parietal, frontal and temporal lobes.

Frontal Lobe

Major areas present in the frontal lobe and their functions are as follows:

- **Motor area:** It is also known as primary motor cortex. The area control muscles of speech and mainly controls fine movements of the fingers and hands.
- **Supplimental motor area:** It lies in the longitudinal fissure. It presents anterior and superior to the premotor area. Along with other outer areas, this area causes altitudinal movements.
- **Premotor areas:** It lies anterior to the motor area. It controls involuntary movements that perform specific tasks.
- **Broca's area:** It is a speech related area causing activation of vocal cords, with movements of mouth and tongue.
- **Prefrontal area:** It lies anterior to area of voluntary eye field and related to important intellectual functions. It helps in concentrating the thoughts, also causes elaboration of thoughts. It also helps in planning the future.
- **Voluntary eye field:** It is located just above the broca's area and is responsible for voluntary eye movements.
- **Area of hand skills:** It is located anterior to 1° motor cortex. It co-ordinates the skillful hand movements.

Parietal lobe

- Major areas of the parietal lobe include;
- **Primary sensory area:** It is associated with general conscious sensations. This receives information from sensations like temperature, touch and pain. This area can judge the texture of material, shapes and forms of objects, weight, pressure, etc.
- **Sensory association area:** It lies behind the primary sensory area and receives stimuli from thalamus, auditory cortex and visual cortex. Recognition of complex objects and complex forms lies with this area.

Occipital lobe

- It contains primary visual area and visual association areas.
- This allows detecting the size, shapes and colours of various objects.
- The secondary visual function is associated with the detection of more complex visual patterns.

Temporal lobe

- It is mainly related to the auditory area.

- The primary and secondary auditory areas of auditory cortex identify the different pitches of sound, judge the intensity of sound and analyses different properties of sound.

Parieto-occipito-temporal association area

- It is associated with intellectual function, reading and learning.
- It is also associated with area of naming objects.

Pre-frontal association area

- It helps the motor area to play complex patterns and sequence of motor movements.
- It is also essential for carrying out prolonged thought processes in the mind.

Limbic association area

- It is associated with behaviour, emotions and motivation.

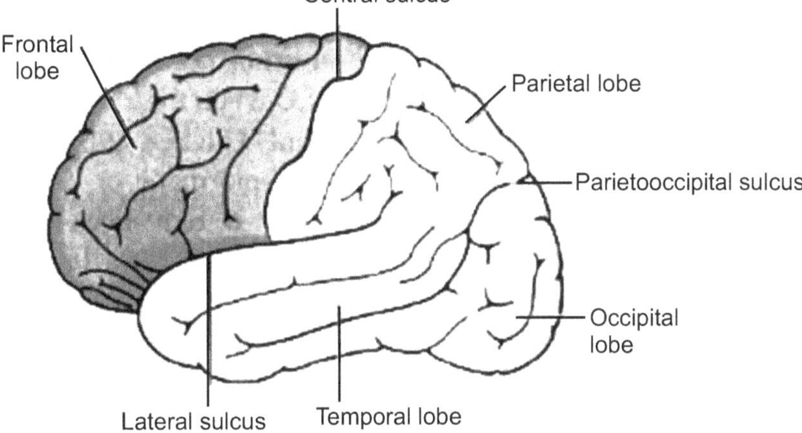

Fig. 1.12: Lobes of the cerebrum

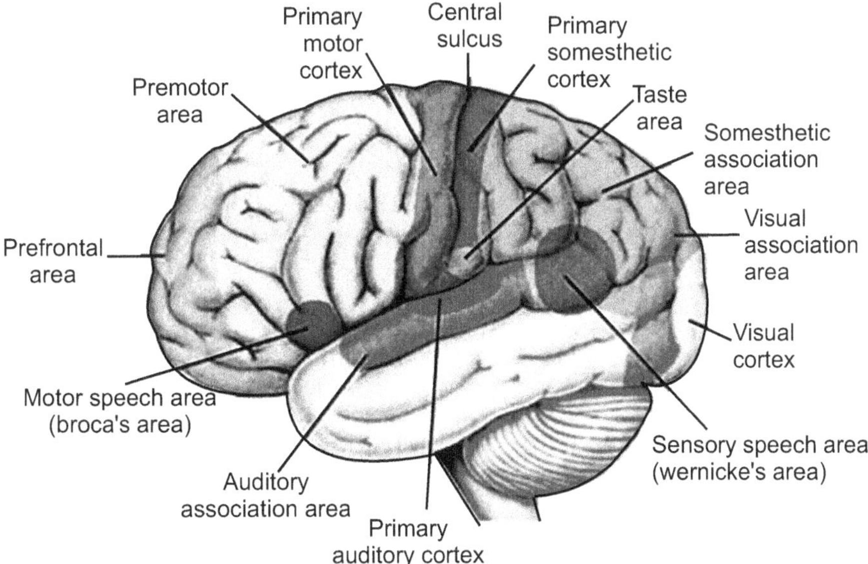

Fig. 1.13: Functional areas of the cerebrum

Functions

- It performs three main activities associated with the cerebral cortex.
- ✓ **Mental activity:** It involves in memory, intelligence, sense of responsibility, thinking, reasoning, moral sense, learning, word formation and interpretation.
- ✓ **Sensory activity:** This involves perception of pain, temperature, touch, sight, hearing, taste and smell.
- ✓ **Motor activity:** It is associated with initiation as well as control of voluntary muscle contraction.

1.14 BASAL GANGLIA

- It is a group of nerve cells (nuclei) present in the medulla of cerebrum.
- Two basal ganglia are:
  - ✓ **Globus pallidus:** It is closer to the thalamus.
  - ✓ **Putamen:** It is closer to the cerebral cortex.
- Together the globus pallidus and putamen forms the lentiform nucleus.
- The third basal ganglia is the caudate nucleus which has two portions-
  - ✓ **Large head**
  - ✓ **Smaller tail**
- Larger head is connected to a smaller tail by a comma-shaped body.
- Together the lentiform nucleus and caudate nuclei are known as corpus striatum.

Functions

- It regulates the initiation and termination of movements.
- It regulates the muscle tone required for specific body movements.
- It also controls subconscious contraction of skeletal muscles

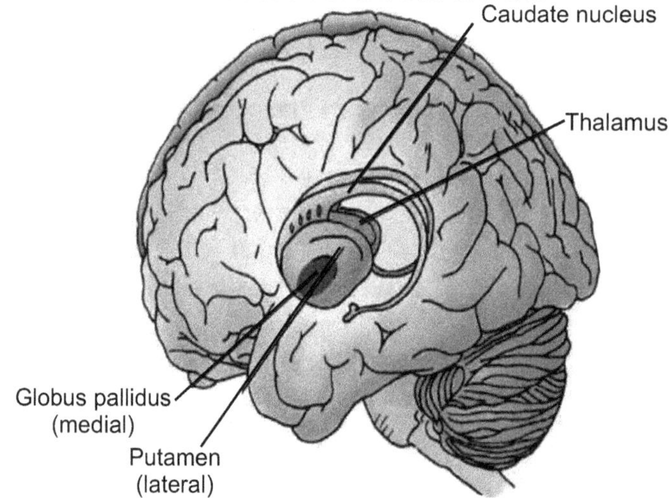

Fig. 1.14: Basal ganglia

1.15 DIENCEPHALON

- It extends from the brain stem to the cerebrum and surrounds the third ventricle.
- The major regions of diencephalon are-
  - ✓ Thalamus
  - ✓ Hypothalamus
  - ✓ Epithalamus

Thalamus

- It measures about 3 cm in length and makes up 80 % of the diencephalon.
- It consists of paired oval masses of gray matter (nerve cells and fibres) situated within the corpus callosum one on each side of the third ventricle.

Functions

- Sensory input from the skin, viscera, special sense organ and pressure is relayed to the thalamus before redistribution to the cerebrum.
- This information is conveyed further to the cerebrum.
- It also plays an important role in regulation of autonomic activities and maintenance of consciousness.

Hypothalamus

- It is a small part of the diencephalon located just below the thalamus, immediately above the pituitary gland.
- It is divided into four main regions.
  - ✓ Mammillary region
  - ✓ Tuberal region
  - ✓ Supraoptic region
  - ✓ Preoptic region

Functions

Control of the autonomic nervous system (ANS)

- It controls and integrates activities of ANS which regulates the contraction of smooth and cardiac muscle along with secretion of many glands.
- It also regulates various visceral activities including regulation of heart rate, movement of food through the gastrointestinal tract and contraction of the urinary bladder.

Production of hormones

- The hypothalamus produces several hormones.

Regulation of emotional and behavioural patterns

- Together with limbic system, the hypothalamus participates in expressions of rage, aggression, pain, pleasure and behavioural patterns related to sexual arousal.

Regulation of eating and drinking

- It regulates the eating and drinking habits.

Control of body temperature

- It controls the body temperature.

Regulation of circadian rhythms and states of consciousness

- It regulates the patterns of awakening and sleep that occurs on a circadian schedule (cycle of about 24 hours).

Epithalamus

- It is a small region, superior and posterior to the thalamus.
- It consists of the pineal gland and habenular nuclei.

- The size of the pineal gland resembles like a small pea.
- It is considered as a part of the endocrine system because it secretes the hormone melatonin.
- More amount of melatonin is liberated during darkness than in light.
- This hormone is thought to promote sleep.

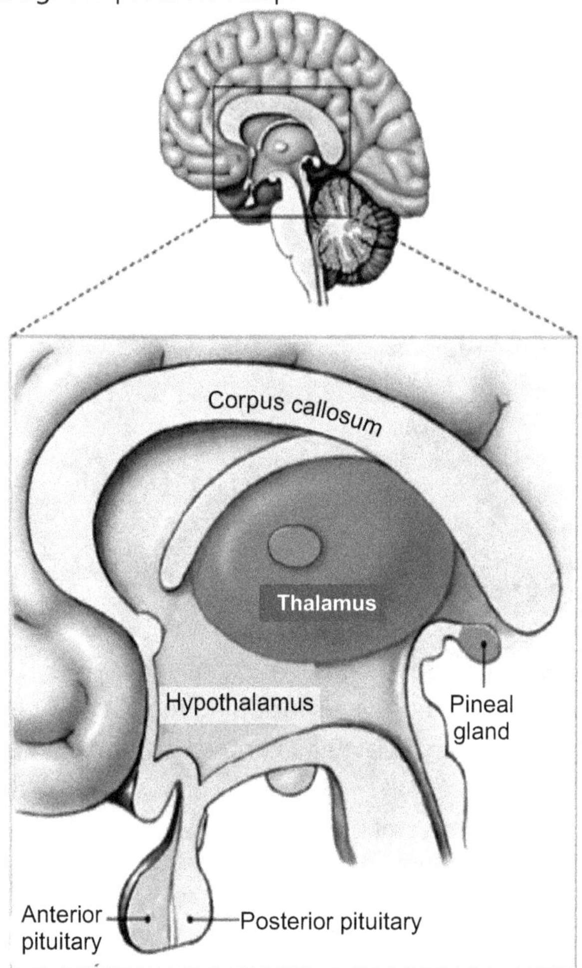

Fig. 1.15: Diencephalon

1.16 CEREBELLUM

- It is the second largest part of the brain.
- It is present posterior to the medulla and pons.
- A deep groove known as the transverse fissure and the tentorium cerebella separates the cerebellum from the cerebrum.
- The shape of the cerebellum is like a butterfly.
- The central constricted area is the vermis and the lateral wings or lobes are the cerebellar hemispheres.

- Each hemisphere consists of three lobes:
  - ✓ Anterior lobe
  - ✓ Posterior lobe
  - ✓ Flocculonodular lobe
- Flocculonodular lobe is concerned with the sense of equilibrium and balance.
- The superficial layer of the cerebellum called as cerebellar cortex, consists of gray matter in a series of slender and parallel ridges called as folia (leaves).
- Deep to the gray matter are tracts called as arbor vitae that look like the branches of a tree.
- In a deep white matter, cerebellar nuclei are present.
- The cerebellum is attached to the brain by three paired cerebellar peduncles.
  - ✓ Inferior cerebellar peduncles
  - ✓ Middle cerebellar peduncles
  - ✓ Superior cerebellar peduncles

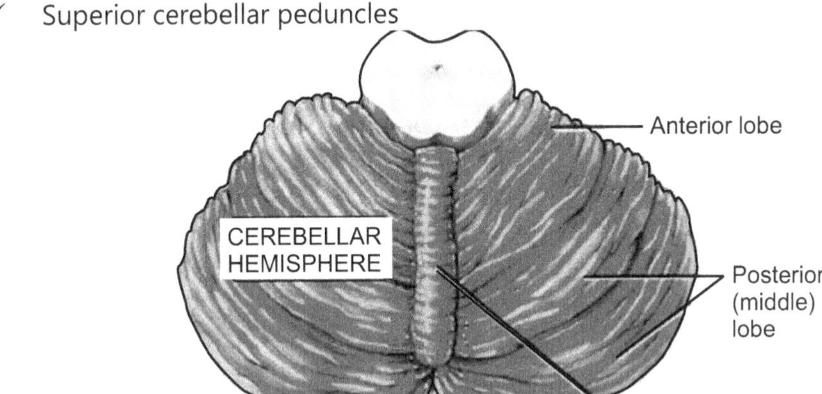

Fig. 1.16 Cerebellum

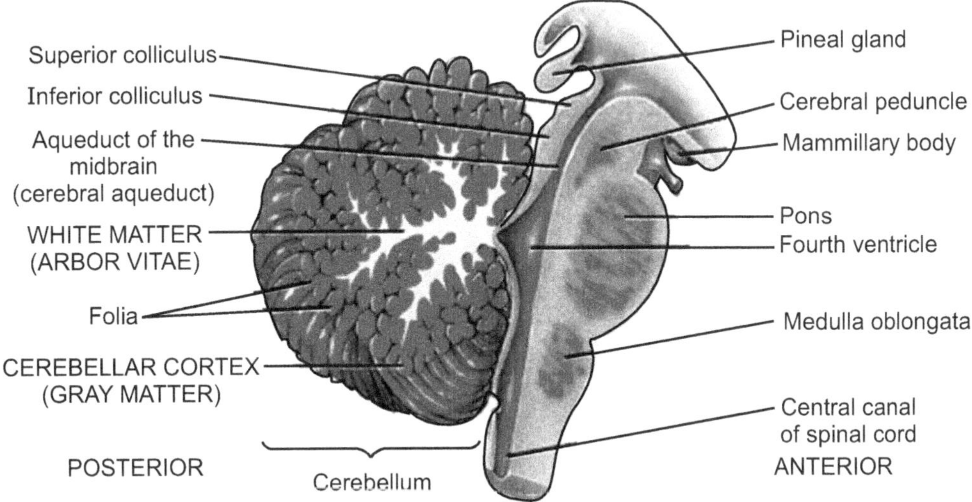

Fig. 1.17: Mid-sagittal section of cerebellum

Functions

- Both voluntary and non-voluntary activities are controlled by the cerebellum.
- It helps the cerebral cortex to co-ordinate patterns of movement involving feet, hands and fingers.
- Posture and equilibrium of the body is controlled by the cerebellum with the help of spinal cord and brain stem.
- It plays an important role in learning and language processing.

1.17 BRAIN STEM

- The brain stem is the lower extension of the brain, located in front of the cerebellum and connected to the spinal cord.
- It is an important center for coordinating eye and facial movements, facial sensation, hearing and balance. The brain stem consists of:
  - ✓ Medulla oblongata
  - ✓ Pons
  - ✓ Midbrain

Medulla oblongata (Medulla)

- It is the lowermost portion of brain stem and superior portion of the spinal cord.
- It is an important centre of the brain as many regulatory centers are located here.
- It contains major centers such as;
- **CVS center:** It regulates rate and force of the heartbeat and the diameter of blood vessels.
- **Medullary rhythmicity area:** It is responsible for adjusting the basic rhythm of breathing
- **Vasomotor center:** It is responsible for monitoring and regulating cardiovascular activities. The vasomotor center is divided into vasoconstrictor area, vasodilator area and the sensory area.
- Other important centers located in the medulla oblongata are the ones that control swallowing, vomiting, coughing, sneezing and hiccupping.
- Medulla also contains nuclei associated with five pairs of cranial nerves.
- **Vestibulocochlear (VIII) nerves:** It is concerned with hearing and equilibrium.
- **Glossopharyngeal (IX) nerves:** It is concerned with swallowing, salivation and taste.
- **Vagus (X) nerves:** It controls vagus and visceral organs
- **Accessory (XI) nerves:** It conveys impulses of movement of head and shoulder.
- **Hypoglossal (XII) nerves:** It conveys nerve impulses related to tongue movements.

Pons

- It is present in front of the cerebellum, just above the medulla oblongata.
- It consists of both nuclei and tracts.
- It is a bridge that connects parts of the brain with one another.
- It contains nuclei for four pairs of cranial nerves.
  - ✓ **Trigeminal nerves (V):** It regulates chewing and sensation of head and face.
  - ✓ **Abducens nerves (VI):** It regulates certain eyeball movements.
  - ✓ **Facial nerves (VII):** It is responsible for sensations of taste, salivation and facial expressions.
  - ✓ **Vestibulocochlear nerves:** It is related to homeostasis.
- Respiratory center is also located in pons which operates along with the rhythmicity area in the medulla.

Mid brain

- It extends from the pons to the diencephalon.
- It also contains nuclei and tracts.
- The anterior part of the midbrain contains a pair of tracts called as cerebral penduncles.
- The posterior part of the midbrain called as tectum contains four rounded elevations.
- Two superior elevations or nuclei known as superior colliculi are responsible for several visual activities.
- Two inferior elevations known as inferior colliculi are responsible for auditory pathways.
- The midbrain also contains other nuclei, left and right substantia nigra, which is large and darkly pigmented.
- It also contains left and right red nuclei, which appears reddish due to their rich blood supply and iron-containing pigment in their neuronal cell body.
- Midbrain is associated with two pairs of cranial nerves.
- **Oculomotor (III) nerves:** It is responsible for eyeball and eyelid movement.
- **Trochlear (IV) nerves:** It innervates the superior oblique muscle of the eye and abducts eyeballs

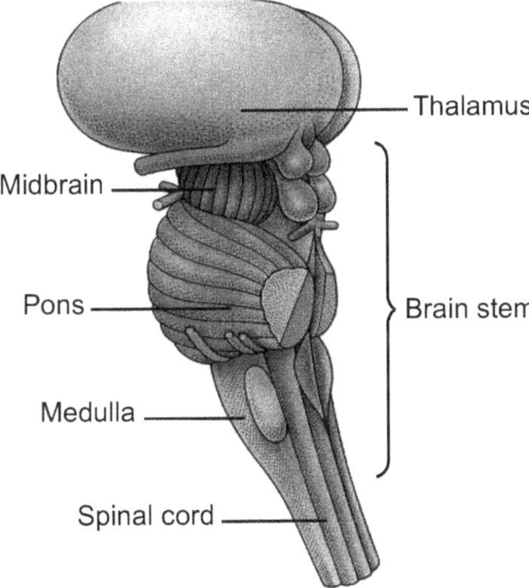

Fig. 1.18: Brain stem

1.18 LIMBIC SYSTEM

- The upper part of the brain stem, the corpus callosum, inner border of the cerebrum and floor of the diencephalon constitute the limbic system.
- The main components of the limbic system are as follows-
- **Cingulate gyrus:** This lies above the corpus callosum.
- **Parahippocompal gyrus:** This lies in the temporal lobe.
- **Hippocampus:** It is a portion of a parahippocompal gyrus present in the temporal lobe.
- **Dentate gyrus:** It lies between the hippocampus and parahippocompal gyrus.
- **Amygdala:** It is composed of numerous neurons located close to the tail of the caudate nucleus.

- **Septal nuclei:** It is located between the septal area formed by the regions under the corpus callosum and the paraterminal gyrus.
- **Mammillary bodies of the hypothalamus:** These are 2 round masses close to the cerebral peduncles.
- **2 nuclei of the thamalus:** The anterior nucleus and the medial nucleus participate in the limbic circuits.
- **Olfactory bulbs:** These are flattened bodies of the olfactory pathway that rest on the cribiform plate.
- **Fornix, stria termilanlis, stria medullarius, medial forebrain bundle and mammilothalamic tract:** These are linked by bundles of interconnecting myelinated axons.

Functions

- It plays a primary role in a range of emotions including pain, pleasure, affection and anger.
- It is also involved in olfaction and memory.
- The hippocampus together with the other part of the cerebrum functions in memory.
- People with damage to certain limbic system structures forget recent events and cannot commit anything to memory.

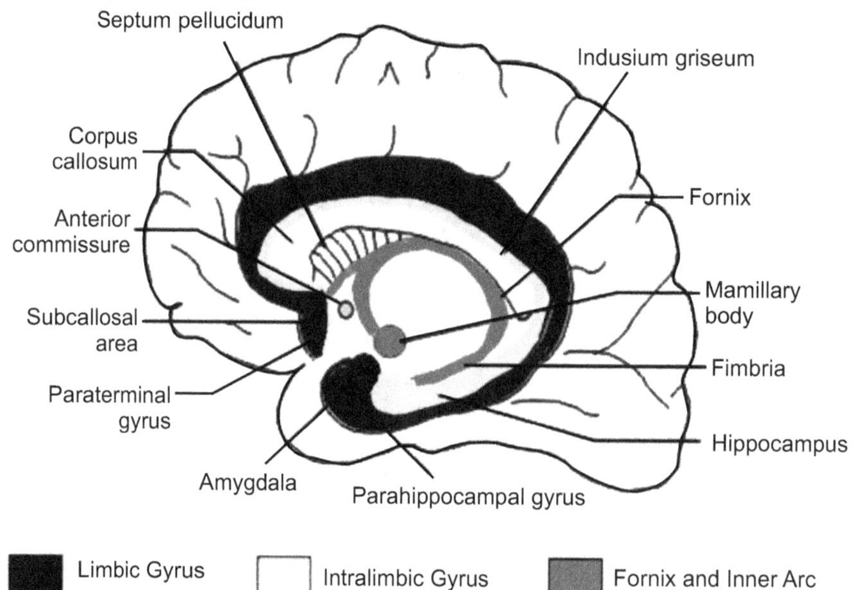

Fig. 1.19: Limbic system

1.19 SPINAL CORD

External Anatomy

- The spinal cord is located within the vertebral column.
- It is roughly cylindrical in shape
- In adults, it extends from the medulla oblongata to the superior border of the second lumbar vertebrae.

- The length of spinal cord ranges from 42-45 cm and diameter is about 2 cm.
- Externally, is shows two enlargements.
  - ✓ **Cervical enlargement:** Superior enlargement extends from the 4th cervical vertebrae to the 1st thoracic vertebrae; nerves to and from the upper limbs arises from the cervical enlargement.
  - ✓ **Lumbar enlargement:** Inferior enlargement extends from the 9th to the 12th thoracic vertebrae; nerves to and from the lower limbs arise from the lumbar enlargement.
- Thirty one pairs of spinal nerves originate from the spinal cord.
- The spinal nerve is connected to the spinal cord by the roots.
- Two types of roots are present:
  - ✓ **Posterior root or dorsal root:** The dorsal or sensory root contains sensory nerve fibers which conducts the nerve impulses from periphery to the spinal cord.
  - ✓ **Anterior root or ventral root:** The ventral or motor root contains motor neurons conducting nerve impulses from the spinal cord to the periphery.

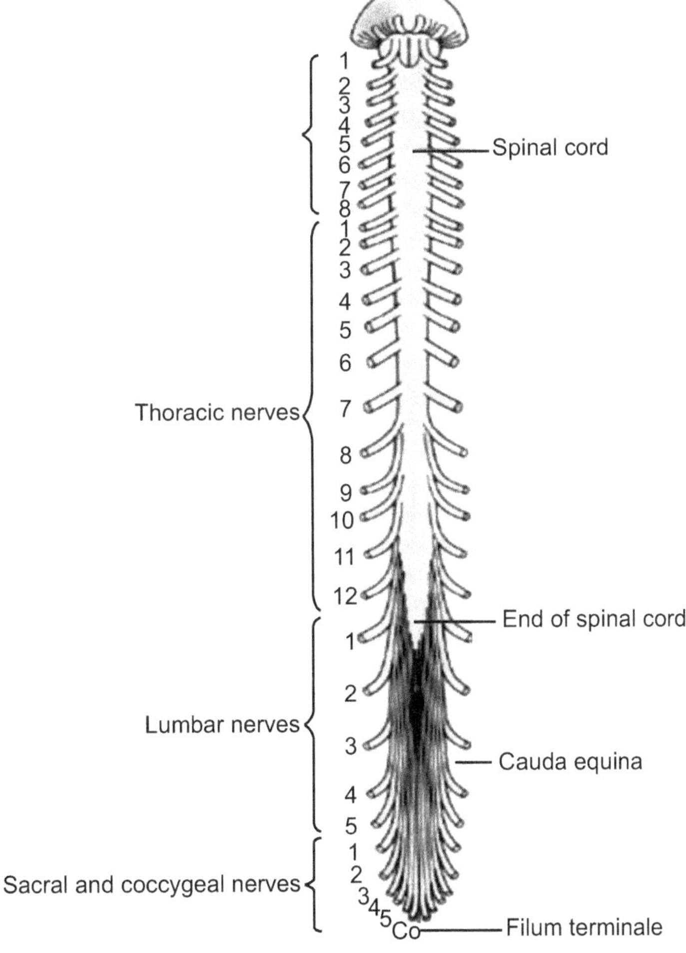

Fig. 1.20: External anatomy of the spinal cord

Internal Anatomy

- The transverse section of spinal cord shows grey matter in the center and white matter surrounding it.
- The shape of the grey matter is like letter 'H' or butterfly shaped.
- The grooves penetrate the white matter of the spinal cord and divide it into right and left sides.
    - ✓ **Anterior median fissure:** Deep grove on anterior (ventral) side
    - ✓ **Posterior median sulcus:** Shallower groove on posterior (dorsal) side
- In the centre of grey matter is a space called the central canal which extends along the entire length of spinal cord.
- The grey matter consists of dendrites, cell bodies of neurons, unmyelinated neurons and neuroglia.
- The white matter consists of bundles of myelinated axons of neurons.
- The grey matter on each side of the spinal cord is divided into regions called as horns.
    - ✓ **Anterior or ventral horns:** Somatic motor nuclei provide nerve (grey) impulses for contraction of skeletal muscles.
    - ✓ **Posterior or dorsal grey horns:** It contains somatic or autonomic sensory nuclei.
- The cell bodies of neurons are located in the grey matter.
- The anterior and posterior grey horns divide the white matter on each side into 3 broad areas called as columns
    - ✓ Anterior (ventral) white columns
    - ✓ Posterior (dorsal) white columns
    - ✓ Lateral white columns

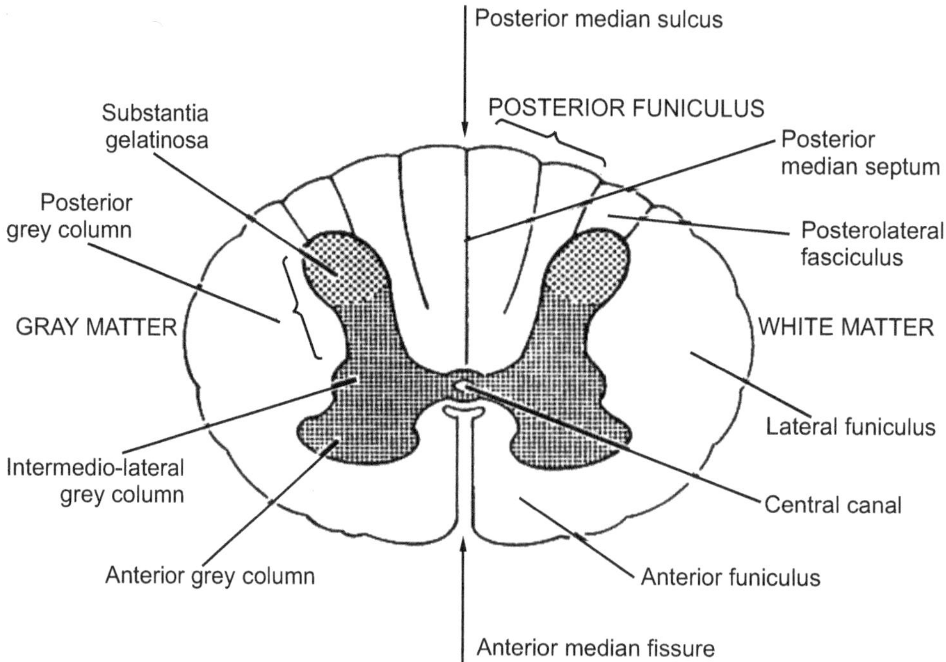

Fig. 1.21: Transverse section of the spinal cord

Division of Spinal Nerves

- There are 31 pairs of spinal nerves originating from the spinal cord.
- According to region they are divided into:
  - Cervical nerves: 8 pairs
  - Thoracic nerves: 12 pairs
  - Lumbar nerves: 5 pairs
  - Sacral nerves: 5 pairs
  - Coccygeal nerves: 1 pair

1.20 REFLEX ARCS

- A reflex arc is a flat, autonomic, unplanned sequence of actions that occurs in response to a particular stimulus.
- When integration takes place in the spinal cord grey matter, the reflex is called as spinal reflex
- If integration occurs in the brain stem it is called as cranial reflex.
- When there is contraction of skeletal muscles it is called as somatic reflexes.
- When there is contraction of smooth muscles, cardiac muscles and glands it is called as autonomic (visceral) reflex.
- The pathway followed by nerve impulses that produce a reflex is called as reflex arc.
- A reflex arc includes the following five functional components:
  - ✓ Sensory receptors
  - ✓ Sensory neuron
  - ✓ Integrating centre
  - ✓ Motor neuron
  - ✓ Effector

Sensory receptor

- The distal end of a sensory neuron (dendrite) serves as a sensory receptor.
- It responds to specific stimulus.
- A change in the internal or external environment produces a graded potential called as receptor potential.
- If a generated potential reaches the polarisation level it will trigger one or more impulses in the sensory neuron.

Sensory neuron

- The nerve impulses propagate from sensory receptor to axon terminals along the axon of the sensory neuron which are located in the grey matter of the spinal cord.

Integrating centre

- One or more regions of the grey matter within the CNS act as an integrating centre.
- The integrating centre is a single synapse between the sensory neuron and the motor neuron.
- The reflex pathway having only one synapse in the CNS is called as monosynaptic reflex arc.

- The integrating centre consists of one or more interneurons which may relay impulses to other interneurons as well as to a motor neuron.
- A polysynaptic reflex arc involves more than one CNS synapse.

Motor neuron

- It carries nerve impulses from the integrating centre to the effector organs.

Effector

- It is the part of body that responds to the motor nerve impulses such as muscle or gland. Its action is called as reflex.
- If the effector is skeletal muscle, the reflex is called as somatic reflex.
- If the effector is smooth muscle, cardiac muscle or gland the reflex is called as an autonomic reflex.

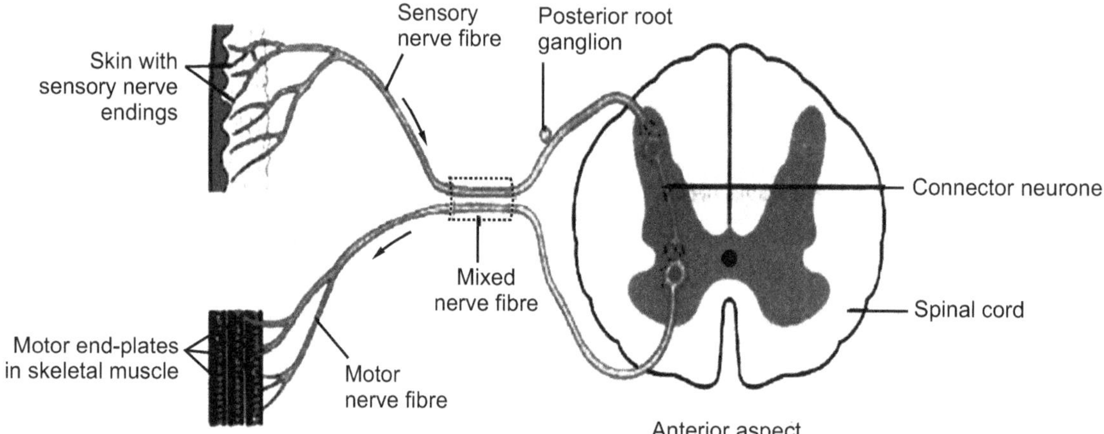

Fig. 1.22: Reflex arc

1.21 DISORDERS OF THE NERVOUS SYSTEM

Multiple sclerosis (MS)

- It is also called as disseminated sclerosis or encephalomyelitis disseminate.
- It is a disease that causes progressive destruction of myelin sheaths of neurons in the central nervous system.
- This myelin sheaths damage disrupts the ability of nervous system to communicate, resulting in a wide range of signs and symptoms, including physical, mental and psychiatric problems.
- It usually appears between the ages of 20 to 40 affecting females twice as often as males.

Epilepsy

- It is characterized by paroxysmal transient disturbances of brain function that may be manifested as episodic impairment or loss of consciousness, abnormal motor phenomena, psychic or sensory disturbances, or perturbation of the autonomic nervous system.

- Symptoms are due to disturbance of the electrical activity of the brain.
- It is characterized by short, recurrent attacks of motor, sensory or psychological malfunctions although it never affects intelligence.
- The attacks are called as epileptic seizures.
- It affects about 1% of the world population.

Cerebrovascular accidents (CVA)

- It is the most common brain disorder; it is also called as stroke or brain attack.
- A CVA is characterized by the various neurological symptoms such as paralysis, loss of sensations that arises from destruction of brain tissue.
- The common causes are intracerebral hemorrhage, emboli (blood clot) and atherosclerosis of the cerebral arteries.

Transient ischemic attacks (TIA)

- It is an episode of temporary cerebral dysfunction caused by impaired blood flow to the brain.
- The symptoms include dizziness, weakness, numbness, or paralysis in a limb or in one side of the body, drooping of one side of the face, headache, slurred speech and a partial loss of vision or double vision.

Alzheimer's disease (AD)

- It is characterized by progressive dementia, loss of reasoning and ability to care for oneself.
- It is a neurodegenerative disorder, primarily affecting the cholinergic neurons in the brain.
- It affects 11 % of population over the age of 65.
- The cause for AD is still unknown, but it may be due to the combination of genetic factors, environmental factors or life style factors.

Brain tumour

- It is an abnormal growth of tissue in the brain that may be malignant or benign.
- The symptoms of a brain tumour depend on its size, location and rate of growth.
- The symptoms are headache, poor balance and coordination, dizziness, double vision, slurred speech, nausea, vomiting, fever, abnormal pulse and breathing rates, personality changes, numbness and weakness of limbs and seizures.

QUESTIONS

Short Answer Questions:
1. Give the classification and functions of nervous system.
2. Explain neuroglia.
3. Give examples of excitatory and inhibitory neurotransmitters.
4. Write a short note on cerebrum.

5. Write a short note on nervous tissue.
6. Write a short note on reflex arc.
7. Write a short note on medulla oblongata.
8. Write a short note on spinal glands.
9. Describe the process of neurotransmission.
10. Draw a neat labeled diagram of spinal cord.
11. Draw a neat labeled diagram of T.S. of spinal cord and explain the internal structure of spinal cord.
12. Enlist various parts of brain and give their functions.

Long Answer Questions:
1. Explain the process of generation of action potentials.
2. Give the internal and external anatomy of spinal cord.
3. Draw well labeled diagram of brain and explain its different parts.
4. Name the various cranial nerves. Explain the internal anatomy of spinal cord and comment on reflex arc.

UNIT II

Chapter **2**...

DIGESTIVE SYSTEM

♦ LEARNING OBJECTIVES ♦

- ❖ To identify the organs of digestive system.
- ❖ To describe the basic processes performed by the digestive system.
- ❖ To describe the structure and function of histological layers of the gastrointestinal tract.
- ❖ To identify the locations of the salivary glands and describe their functions.
- ❖ To describe the structure and functions of the tongue.
- ❖ To describe the parts of a typical tooth, and different types of teeth.
- ❖ To study composition and function of saliva.
- ❖ To describe the location and function of the pharynx.
- ❖ To describe the location, anatomy and physiology of the esophagus.
- ❖ To describe the three phases of deglutition.
- ❖ To describe the location, anatomy and physiology of the stomach.
- ❖ To describe the phases of mechanical and chemical digestion in stomach.
- ❖ To describe the location, anatomy and function of the pancreas.
- ❖ To describe the composition and function of pancreatic juice.
- ❖ To describe the location, anatomy and function of the liver and gall bladder.
- ❖ To describe the composition and function of bile.
- ❖ To describe the location, anatomy and functions of the small and large intestine.
- ❖ To describe the composition and function of intestinal juice.
- ❖ To describe the phases of digestion.

2.1 INTRODUCTION

Digestion is the process of breaking down of larger food molecules into smaller molecules with the help of digestive enzymes and acid. The digestive system contributes to homeostasis by breaking down food into forms that can be absorbed and used by body cells. It also absorbs water, vitamins, minerals and eliminates wastes from the body. Most of the food material that we eat is available in complex form and need to convert into simpler form. The medical branch that deals with the structure, function, diagnosis and treatment of diseases of the stomach and intestines is called as gastroenterology.

Digestive system is made up of

- **Gastrointestinal tract or alimentary canal:** It consists of Mouth, Pharynx, Oesophagus, Stomach, Small Intestine and Large Intestine.

(2.1)

- **Accessory structures:** It consists of Teeth, Tongue, Salivary glands, Liver, Gall bladder and Pancreas.

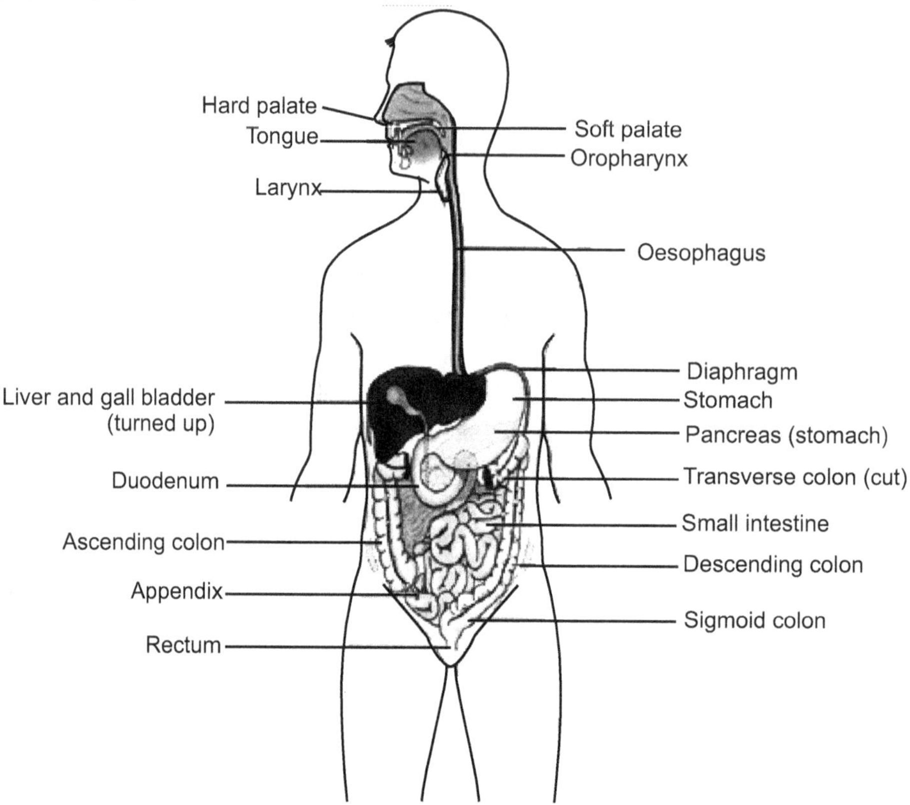

Fig. 2.1: Digestive system

2.2 DIGESTIVE PROCESSES

Digestive system performs five basic activities:

- ✓ **Ingestion:** Taking food into the mouth (eating)
- ✓ **Movement of food:** Passage of food along the gastrointestinal tract (GIT)
- ✓ **Digestion:** Breakdown of food by both chemical and mechanical processes
- ✓ **Absorption:** The passage of digested food from GIT into the cardiovascular and lymphatic system for distribution to cells
- ✓ **Defecation:** The elimination of indigestible substances from the GIT.

2.3 HISTOLOGY OF GIT

- The wall of GI tract from the esophagus to anal canal has some basic arrangement of tissues.
- It consists of 4 layers or tunics from the inside to outside of tract.
  - ✓ **Mucosa:** It is the inner lining of tract. It consists of three layers i.e. Epithelium, Lamina propria and Muscularis mucosae
  - ✓ **Submucosa:** It is the layer which is present above the mucosa. It consists of areolar connective tissue that binds the mucosa to the third layer, the muscularis.
  - ✓ **Muscularis:** It is the layer which is present above the submucosa layer.
  - ✓ **Serosa:** It is the outermost layer of GIT.

2.4 MOUTH

- It is also called as the oral or buccal cavity.
- It is formed by the cheeks, hard and soft palates and tongue.
- Forming the lateral structure (walls) of the oral cavity are the cheeks.
- The anterior portions of the cheeks terminate in the superior and inferior lips.
- The lips are fleshy folds surrounding the opening of the mouth.
- They are covered on the outside by skin and on inside by a mucus membrane.
- The hard palate is the anterior portion of the roof of mouth.
- The soft palate is the posterior portion of the roof of mouth.

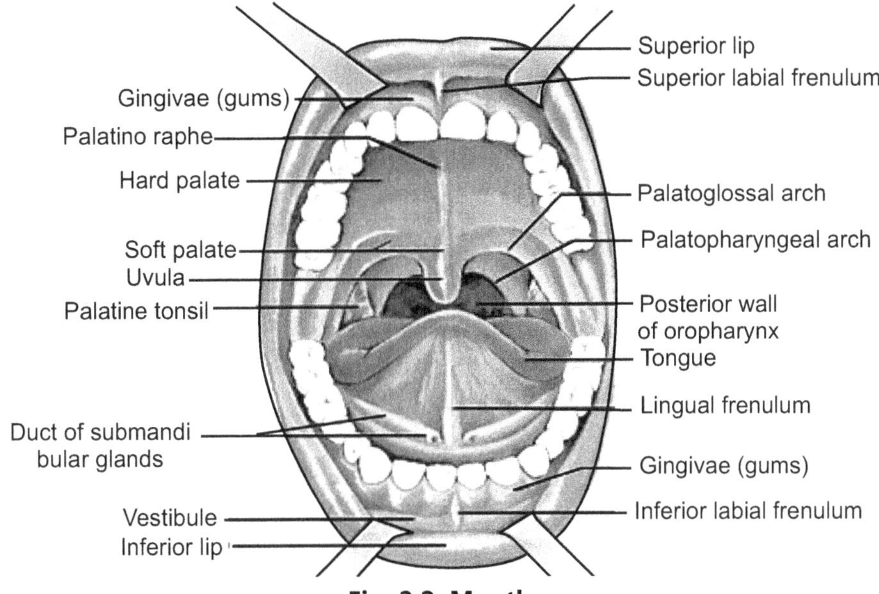

Fig. 2.2: Mouth

2.5 TONGUE

- The tongue, together with other associated muscles forms the floor of the oral cavity.
- It is an accessory structure of the digestive system composed of skeletal muscle covered with mucous membrane.
- The upper surface and sides of tongue are covered with papillae, projection of lamina propria covered with epithelium.
  - ✓ **Filiform papillae:** It is whitish in colour and has no taste buds.
  - ✓ **Fungiform papillae:** More numerous near the tip of tongue, reddish dot and most of them contain taste buds.
  - ✓ **Circumvallate papillae:** All of them contain taste buds.

Function of tongue

1. Mastication (Chewing)
2. Deglutition (Swallowing)
3. Speech
4. Taste

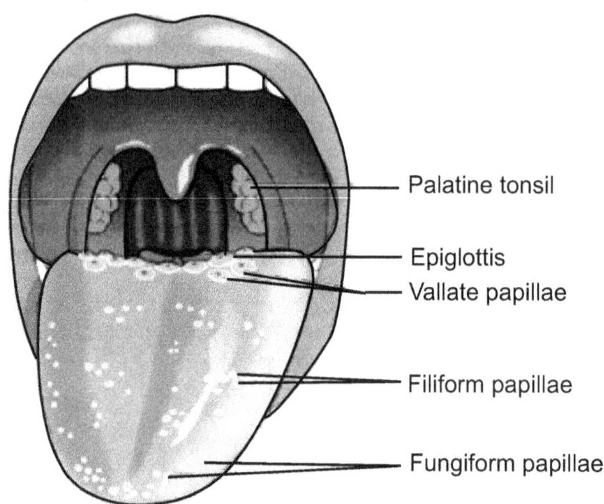

Fig. 2.3: Tongue

2.6 TEETH

- The teeth (dentes) are accessory structure of the digestive system located in sockets of the alveolar processes of the mandible (lower jaw bone) and maxillae (upper jaw bone).
- The alveolar processes are covered by gum.
- The visible portion of tooth above the gums is called as crown.
- The socket embedded portion is called as root.
- Teeth are made up of a calcified connective tissue called as dentin.
- This dentin is covered by a layer of enamel consisting of calcium phosphate and calcium carbonate.
- Enamel being very hard, protect the teeth from wear of chewing and is also acid resistant.
- Each person has two sets of teeth.
  - ✓ **Falling out set of teeth or Deciduous teeth**
  - ✓ **Permanent set of teeth**
- Between the age of 6 to 12 years all deciduous teeth/milk or baby teeth are lost and are replaced by permanent teeth.
- The permanent set of teeth consists of 32 teeth.

Shapes of permanent teeth

- There are four shapes of permanent teeth.
  - ✓ Molar
  - ✓ Premolar
  - ✓ Canine
  - ✓ Incisor
- Premolar and molar teeth are broad, with flat surfaces and are used for grinding or chewing of food.
- Incisors and molar teeth are the cutting teeth and are used for biting off pieces of food.

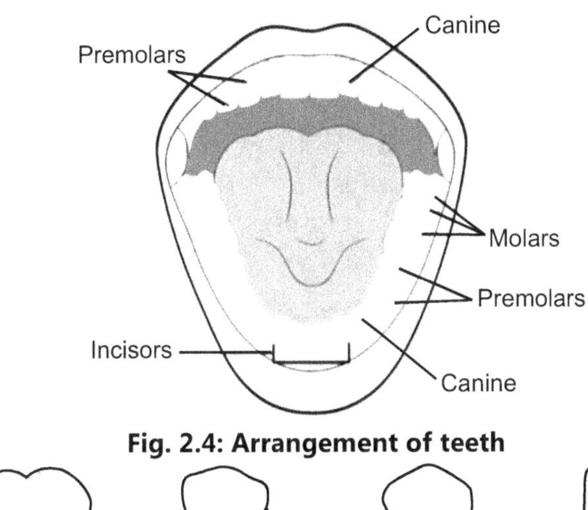

Fig. 2.4: Arrangement of teeth

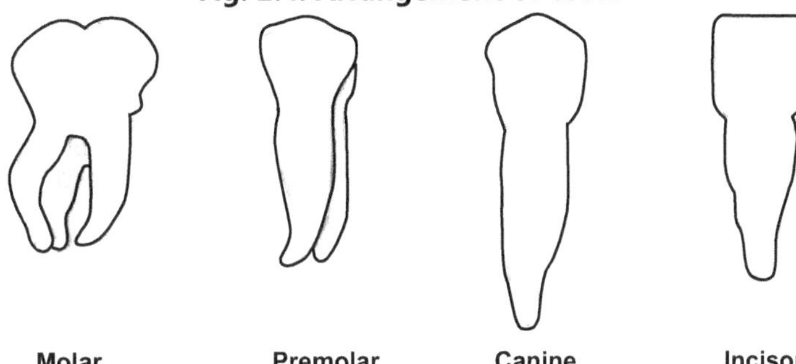

Fig. 2.5: Shapes of permanent teeth

Parts of Teeth

- There are three parts of teeth:
  - ✓ The crown
  - ✓ The root
  - ✓ The neck
- In the centre of the tooth is the pulp cavity containing blood vessels, lymph vessels and nerves.

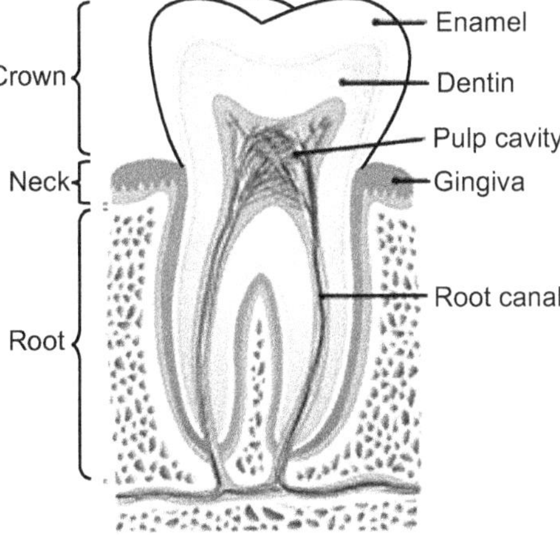

Fig. 2.6: Teeth

2.7 SALIVARY GLANDS

- The salivary gland releases a secretion called as saliva into the oral cavity.
- Three pairs of salivary glands are present in the mouth.
  - ✓ **Parotid glands:** They are present inferior and anterior to the ears. They secrete their secretion in the oral cavity by parotid duct. It is the largest salivary gland.
  - ✓ **Submandibular glands:** These are present in the posterior part of the floor of mouth, beneath the base of tongue. They secrete their secretions into oral cavity by submandibular ducts.
  - ✓ **Sublingual glands:** It is the smallest of salivary glands and present beneath the tongue.

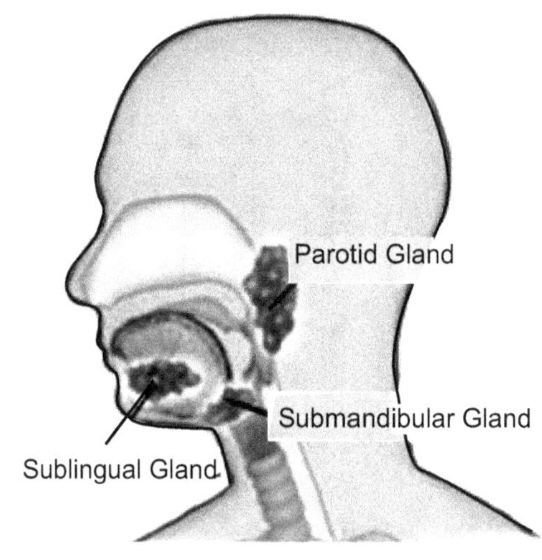

Fig. 2.7: Salivary glands

2.8 SALIVA

- It consists of 99.5% water and 0.5% solutes.
- Among the solutes are ions including sodium, potassium, chloride, bicarbonate and phosphate, some gases various organic substances including urea and uric acid, mucus, immunoglobulin A, lysozyme enzyme and amylase enzyme.
- About 1 to 1.5 liters saliva is secreted every day.
- It is slightly acidic in nature (pH 6.35 to 6.85).
- It is viscous and colourless in nature.

Functions of saliva

- **Cleaning:** It helps in cleaning the mouth and teeth; keeping them free from debris and prevents the excessive growth of bacteria.
- **Moistening and lubrication:** It lubricates and moistens the soft part of mouth, keeping it pliable for speech.

- **Excretion:** Many organic substances like urea and inorganic substances like mercury, lead and many drugs are excreted in the saliva.
- **Chemical digestion of polysaccharides:** It contains the enzyme amylase that brings about the breakdown of complex sugars like starch.
- **Lubrication of food:** It produces moistening and lubrication of dry food entering into the mouth.

2.9 PHARYNX

- When food is first swallowed, it passes from mouth into the pharynx (throat), a funnel shaped tube of about 13 cm long.
- It starts at the internal nares to the esophagus posteriorly and the larynx anteriorly.
- Its wall is composed of skeletal muscle and is lined with mucous membrane.
- It acts as a passageway for the air and food.

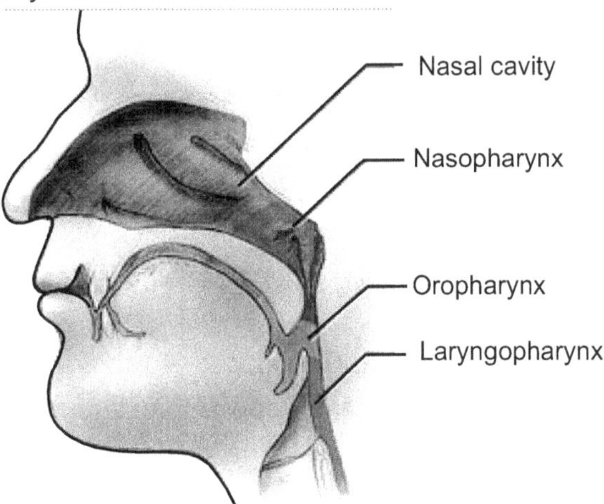

Fig. 2.8: Pharynx

- It is divided into three parts.
  - ✓ **Nasopharynx:** It is the superior portion of larynx and is important for respiration. It moves the bolus from oropharynx to laryngopharynx and into the oesophagus.
  - ✓ **Oropharynx:** The intermediate portion of the pharynx is the oropharynx. It lies posterior to the oral cavity.
  - ✓ **Laryngopharynx:** The inferior portion of pharynx is the laryngopharynx or hypo pharynx, begins at the level of hyoid bone. It opens into the esophagus posteriorly and the larynx (voice box) anteriorly.
- Oropharynx and laryngopharynx are common for both respiratory and digestive system.

2.10 ESOPHAGUS

- It is a collapsible muscular tube of about 25 cm long and 2 cm in diameter that lies posterior to the trachea.

- It is continuous with the pharynx and just below the diaphragm it joins the stomach.
- The upper and lower ends of oesophagus are closed by sphincters.
  - ✓ **Upper esophageal sphincter**: It regulates the movement of food from the pharynx into the oesophagus.
  - ✓ **Lower esophageal sphincter:** It regulates the movement of food from the oesophagus into the stomach.

2.11 SWALLOWING (DEGLUTITION)

- It is a complex but fast process which is completed within few seconds.
- It is divided into three stages;

Buccal swallowing

  - ✓ The buccal swallowing is under voluntary control.
  - ✓ Once mouth is closed the bolus is collected on the upper surface of tongue.
  - ✓ By the upward and downwards movement of tongue the bolus is brought to oropharynx.

Pharyngeal swallowing

  - ✓ Since, the pharynx communicates with both esophagus and trachea, the next step is to allow the bolus to enter the esophagus, avoiding the air passages.
  - ✓ The bolus is forced back upon the epiglottis which closes the laryngeal orifice.
  - ✓ This makes the food pass to the laryngopharynx and then into the esophagus.

Esophageal swallowing

  - ✓ The esophagus at rest is relaxed but it is closed at top and bottom by sphincters.
  - ✓ The lower sphincter is weaker than the upper sphincter.
  - ✓ The motor activity of esophagus is under the control of vagus nerve.
  - ✓ Once, the food is within the esophagus through the peristaltic movements the food is brought into the stomach.

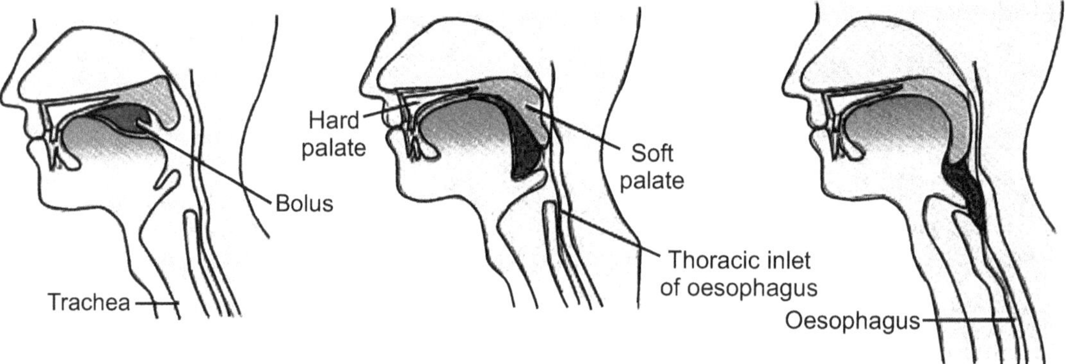

Fig. 2.9: Phases of swallowing

2.12 STOMACH

- It is an enlargement of gastro-intestinal tract and is nearly a J shaped organ.

- It is a connecting organ between esophagus and duodenum.
- The stomach can be divided into four main areas.
- **The Cardia:** It is located near superior opening of the stomach.
- **The Fundus:** It is a rounded portion present superior and to the left of cardia.
- **The Body:** It is the large central portion of the stomach and present inferior to the fundus.
- **The Pylorus:** It is located below the body of stomach. The region of the stomach that connects to the duodenum is the pylorus.
- It has two parts.
  - ✓ **Pyloric antrum:** It connects to the body of stomach.
  - ✓ **Pyloric canal:** It connects to the duodenum called as pyloric canal which contains the pyloric sphincter.
- The concave border of stomach is called as lesser curvature.
- The convex border of stomach is called as greater curvature.

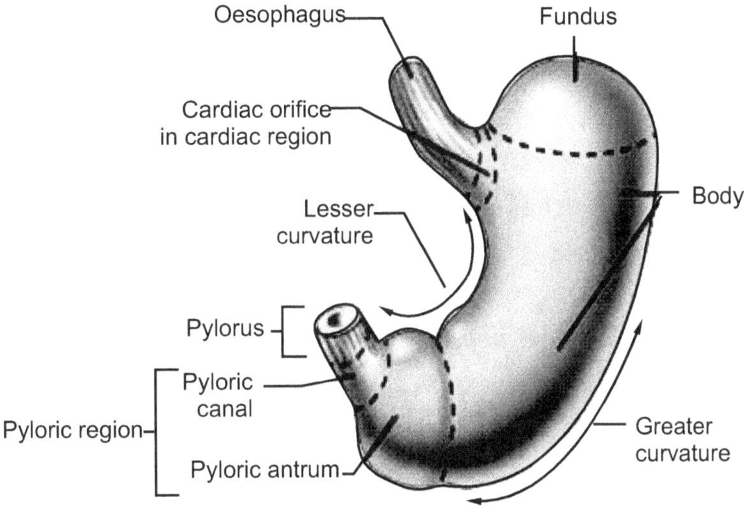

Fig. 2.10: Stomach

Functions of Stomach

- It acts as a reservoir of food. The stomach can distend with accumulation of food intake.
- With the peristaltic movement it causes the mixing of food with the gastric juice.
- The mucosal lining of stomach is responsible for absorbing some quantity of water, alcohol, glucose to the blood stream.
- It causes secretion of about 1 to 2 litres of gastric juice every day.
- The gastric lipase possesses lipolytic activity.
- Pepsin causes chemical breakdown of protein to proteases and peptones.
- The mucus cell secretes mucus and prevents mechanical injury to stomach.

- The strong acidic pH of hydrochloric acid kills the bacteria in food and provides protection.
- Stomach forms the intrinsic factors which is needed for the absorption of vitamin B_{12}.
- The presence of cardiac sphincter inhibits reflux acid from stomach to oesophagus.

Histology of Stomach

- The wall of stomach is composed of same basic layers as that of gastro-intestinal tract, with some modifications.
- The surface of the mucosa is made up of simple columnar epithelial cells called as surface mucous cells.
- The mucosa contains two more layers such as lamina propria made up of areolar connective tissue and muscularis mucosae made up of smooth muscle.
- Epithelial cells of mucosa layer extend down into the lamina propria layer, where they form columns of secretory cells called as gastric glands.
- Numerous gastric glands open into the bottom of narrow channels called as gastric pits.
- The secretions of the gastric glands flow into each gastric pit and then enter into the lumen of the stomach.
- The gastric glands contain three types of gland cells that secrete their secretions into the stomach lumen such as; mucous neck cells, parietal cells and chief cells.
- The function of surface mucous cells and mucous neck cells is to secrete the mucus.
- The function of Parietal cells is to production of intrinsic factor (needed for absorption of vitamin B_{12}) and hydrochloric acid.
- The chief cells secrete enzymes pepsinogen and gastric lipase.
- The combined secretions of the mucous cells, parietal cells and chief cells form the gastric juice.
- Near about 2000–3000 ml gastric juice is secreted daily.
- The enteroendocrine cell (G cell) in the gastric glands is mainly located in the pyloric antrum and secretes the hormone gastrin into the bloodstream responsible for secretion of several aspects of gastric activity.
- Three different layers are present deep to the mucosa.
- **Submucosa:** It is composed of areolar connective tissue.
- **Muscularis:** It consists of three different layers of smooth muscle.
    - ✓ Outer longitudinal layer
    - ✓ Middle circular layer
    - ✓ Inner oblique layer.
- **Serosa:** It is composed of simple squamous epithelium and areolar connective tissue.

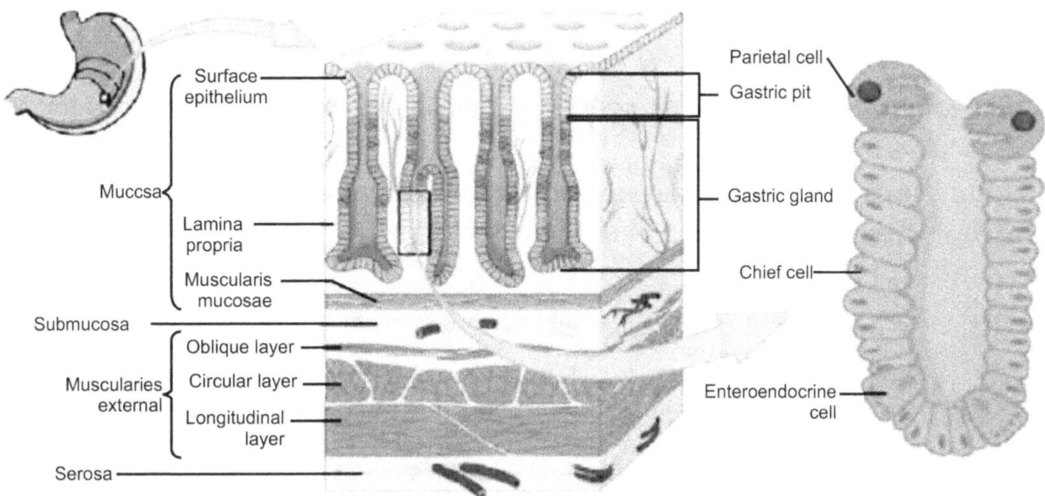

Fig. 2.11: Histology of Stomach

2.13 MECHANICAL AND CHEMICAL DIGESTION IN STOMACH

- After the entry of food inside the stomach mild, flowing, peristaltic movements called as mixing waves passes over the stomach after every 15 to 25 seconds.

- These mixing waves produces maceration of food, mix it with the secretions of gastric glands and convert it into a liquid called as chyme.

- As soon as digestion proceeds in the stomach, more energetic mixing waves starts at the body of stomach and strengthen as they reach the pylorus region of the stomach.

- The pyloric sphincter normally remains closed but as food reaches the pylorus, each mixing wave forces about 3 ml of chyme into the duodenum through the pyloric sphincter, the phenomenon is known as gastric emptying.

- Most of the chyme juice is forced back into the body of stomach, where the mixing process continues.

- The next wave pushes the chyme forward again and forces a little more into the duodenum.

- These forward and backward movements of the gastric contents are responsible for maximum mixing in the stomach.

- After that, digestion of the food by salivary amylase continues. But, the churning action mixes the chyme with acidic gastric juice, inactivating salivary amylase enzyme and activating lipase enzyme, which causes digestion of triglycerides into fatty acids and diglycerides.

- The parietal cells secrete hydrogen ions (H^+) and chloride ions (Cl^-) separately into the stomach lumen; the resultant net effect is secretion of hydrochloric acid (HCl) (Figure 2.13).

- The proton pumps powered by H^+/K^+ ATPase actively transport H^+ into the lumen while allows entry of potassium ions (K^+) into the cell (Fig. 2.13).
- At the same time, Cl^- and K^+ diffuse out into the lumen through Cl^- and K^+ channels in the apical membrane.
- The enzyme carbonic anhydrase, present in the parietal cells, forms carbonic acid (H_2CO_3) from water (H_2O) and carbon dioxide (CO_2).
- As carbonic acid undergoes dissociation, it provides a source of H^+ for the proton pumps but on the other hands it also produces bicarbonate ions (HCO_3^-).
- As HCO_3^- builds up in the cytosol, it exits the parietal cell in exchange for Cl^- via. Cl^-/HCO_3^- antiporters in the basolateral membrane (present next to the lamina propria) and HCO_3^- diffuses into the nearby blood capillaries.
- This condition is called as alkaline tide of bicarbonate ions that enters the blood stream after a meal may be large to increase the blood pH slightly and make the urine more alkaline.
- The HCl secretion by parietal cells can be stimulated by numerous source:
  - ✓ Acetylcholine released by parasympathetic neurons
  - ✓ Gastrin secreted by G cells
  - ✓ Histamine released by mast cells in the nearby lamina propria
- The strong acidic fluid of the stomach kills many micro-organisms in the food.
- HCl also denatures (unfolds) proteins in food and stimulates the secretion of hormones that promote the flow of bile and pancreatic juice.
- Enzymatic digestion of proteins also begins in the stomach.
- Pepsin is protein-digesting enzyme present in the stomach, is secreted by the chief cells.
- Enzyme pepsin breaks down a protein chain of many amino acids into smaller peptide fragments in the acidic environment of the stomach (pH 2) and it inactive at a higher pH.
- Other enzyme present in the stomach is gastric lipase that splits the short-chain triglycerides in fat molecules into fatty acids and monoglycerides at the acidic pH 5-6.
- Only a minor amount of nutrients are absorbed in the stomach because the epithelial cells are impermeable to most of the materials.
- Whereas, the mucous cells of the stomach absorb some water, ions and short chain fatty acids, as well as certain drugs and alcohol.
- Within 2 to 4 hours after eating a meal, the stomach empties its contents into the duodenum.
- Foods rich in carbohydrate spend the least time in the stomach; high-protein foods remain longer, and emptying of stomach is very slow after eating a fatty meal.

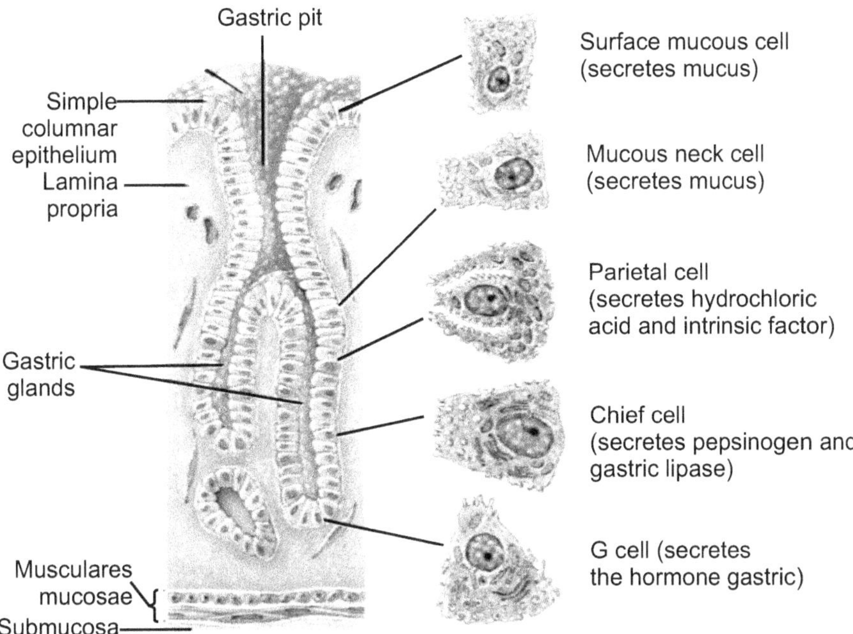

Fig. 2.12: Different types of cells present in the stomach mucosa

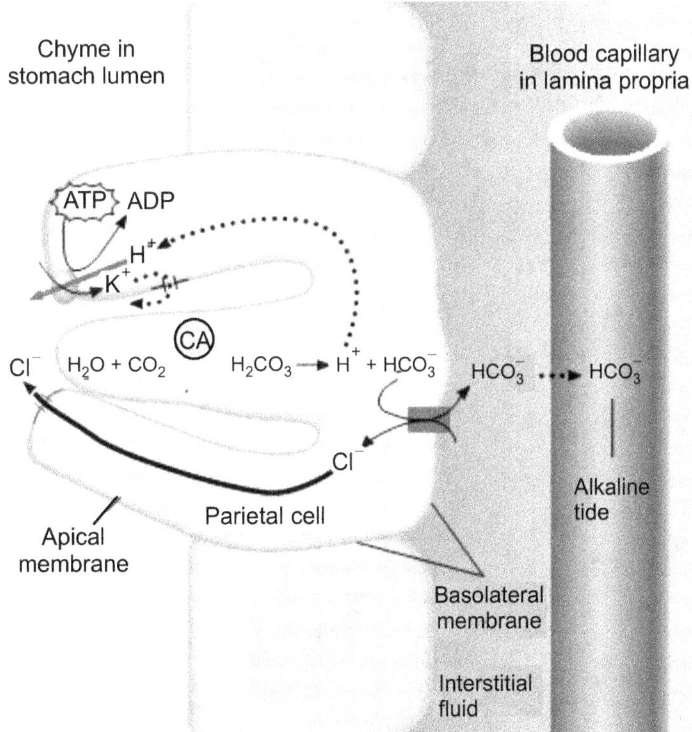

Fig. 2.13: Secretion of HCl by parietal cells in the stomach

2.14 GASTRIC JUICE

- It is clear, colourless fluid, isotonic to blood and acidic in nature.
- About two liters of gastric juice are secreted daily by secretory glands in the mucosa.
- It consists of:
  - ✓ **Water:** It is secreted by gastric glands.
  - ✓ **Mineral salts:** It is secreted by gastric glands.
  - ✓ **Mucus:** It is secreted by goblet cells in the glands.
  - ✓ **Hydrochloric acid:** It is secreted by parietal cells in gastric glands.
  - ✓ **Intrinsic factor:** It is secreted by parietal cells in gastric glands.
  - ✓ **Inactive enzyme pepsinogen:** It is secreted by chief cells in the glands.

Functions of Gastric juice

- **Water:** It liquefies the swallowed food.
- **Hydrochloric acid:** It activates pepsinogen to pepsin which hydrolyses the proteins to polypeptides and kills the ingested micro-organism.
- **Intrinsic factors:** These are essential for absorption of vitamin B_{12} from the ileum.
- **Mucus:** It prevents mechanical injury to stomach wall by lubricating the contents.

2.15 SMALL INTESTINE

- The small intestine is continuous with the stomach at the pyloric sphincter and leads into the large intestine at the ileocaecal valve.
- It is thin and long tube.
- The diameter is about 1.5 inches and 5 meters long and lies in the abdominal cavity surrounded by large intestine.
- In small intestine the chemical digestion of food is completed and most of the absorption of nutrients takes place.
- It is divided into three portions.
  - ✓ **The duodenum:** It is the shortest region. It starts at the pyloric sphincter of the stomach and extends upto the jejunum. It is 25 cm long.
  - ✓ **The jejunum:** It is the middle portion. It extends from duodenum to the ileum. It is 1 m long.
  - ✓ **The ileum:** It is the terminal portion. It is 2 cm long. It extends from the jejunum and joins the large intestine at ileocaecal junction having ileocaecal sphincters.

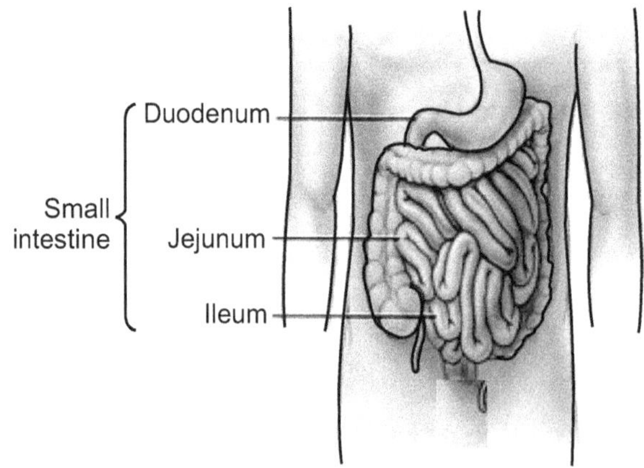

Fig. 2.14: Small intestine

Functions of small intestine

- Onward movement of its contents by peristalsis which is increased by Parasympathetic Nervous System (PNS) stimulation.
- Secretion of intestinal juice, also increased by PNS.
- Completion of chemical digestion of carbohydrates, proteins and fats in the enterocytes of villi.
- Secretion of hormones cholecystokinin (CCK) and secretin.
- Absorption of vitamins.

Histology

- The wall of small intestine is made up of four layers.
  - ✓ Mucosa
  - ✓ Sub-mucosa
  - ✓ Muscularis
  - ✓ Serosa
- The innermost mucosa forms numerous fingers like projections and they increase the surface area of epithelium thereby providing large surface area available for absorption.
- The mucosal epithelium is made up of simple columnar epithelium.
- Around four types of cells are present in the simple columnar epithelium.
  - ✓ **The absorptive cells with brush border of microvilli:** These microvilli greatly increase the surface area for absorption and therefore larger amount of digested material (nutrients) can diffuse into the absorptive cells of intestinal wall. Several digestive enzymes are linked with microvilli.
  - ✓ **Goblet cells:** These are present in the epithelium which secretes the mucus.
  - ✓ **Enteroendocrine cells:** Three types of enteroendocrine cells are found in the mucosa of gastrointestinal tract. S cells: Secrets secretin, K cells: Secrets Glucose dependent insulinotropic peptide and CCK cells: Secrets cholecystokinin.
  - ✓ **Paneth cells:** It is found in the deepest parts of the intestinal gland. The Paneth cells are phagocytic in nature and secrete bactericidal enzyme lysosomes.
- Submucosa of duodenum also contains duodenal glands which secrete alkaline mucus that helps neutralize gastric acid in the chyme.

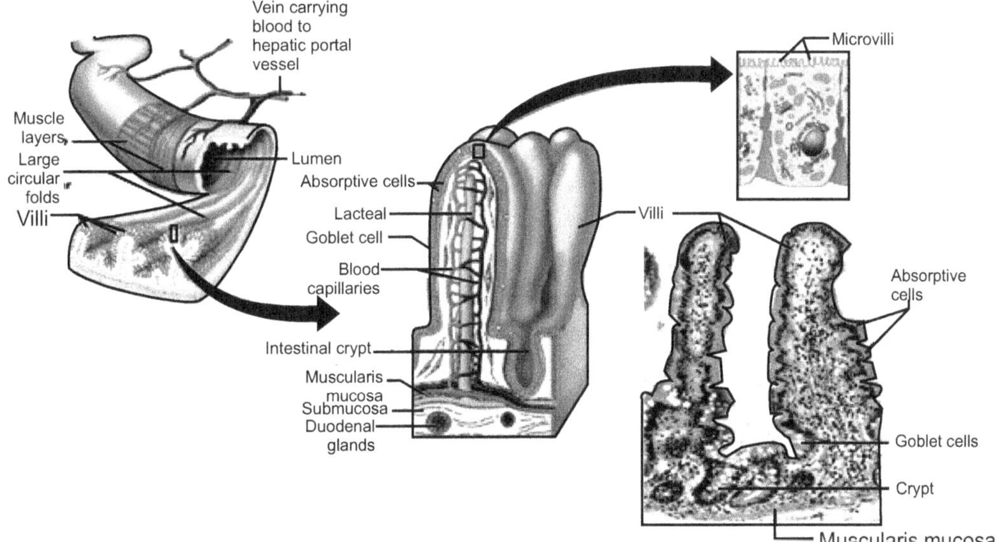

Fig. 2.15: Histology of small intestine

2.16 INTESTINAL JUICE

- About 1 to 2 liters of intestinal juice is secreted every day.
- It is a clear yellow fluid, alkaline in nature (pH 7.6 - 8.0).
- It consists of water, mucus and mineral salts.
- The intestinal juice contains several digestive enzymes.
- These includes;
    - ✓ **Peptidases:** It splits peptides to amino acid.
    - ✓ **Amylase:** It splits starch to maltose.
    - ✓ **Lactase and sucrose:** It splits disaccharides to monosaccharides.
    - ✓ **Maltose:** It splits maltose to glucose.
    - ✓ **Lipase:** It splits glycerides to lower glycerides, fatty acid and glycerol.

2.17 MECHANICAL DIGESTION IN SMALL INTESTINE

- There are two types of movements of small intestine.

Segmentation
- These are rhythmic alternating contraction and relaxation of small intestine.
- These movements mix the chyme with the digestive juices and bring the food particles into contact with mucosa for absorption.

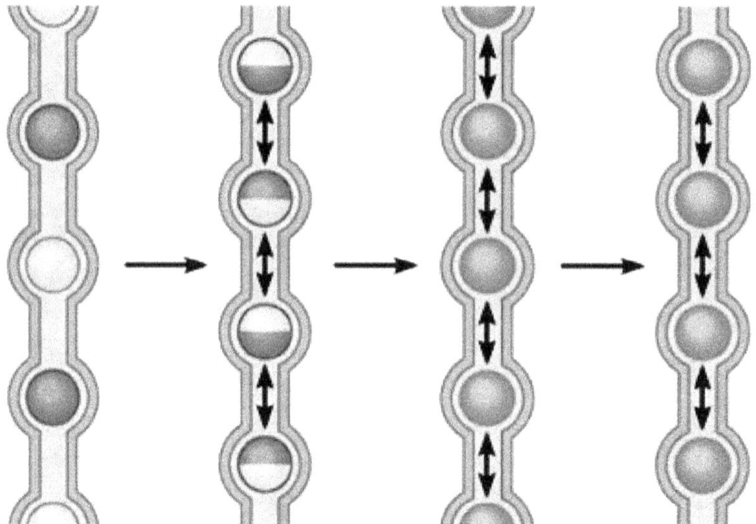

Fig. 2.16: Segmentation in small intestine

Peristalsis
- Entry of food into the small intestine stimulates the stretch receptors and stretch receptors convey information to the CNS.
- The parasympathetic division (PNS) stimulates contraction of intestine and the sympathetic division (SNS) decreases motility of small intestine.
- Therefore, segmentation is myogenic in nature, i.e. it is the property of the smooth muscle. It does not depend on nervous mechanism. Whereas, the peristaltic movements are neurogenic i.e. it is carried out with the help of SNS and PNS.

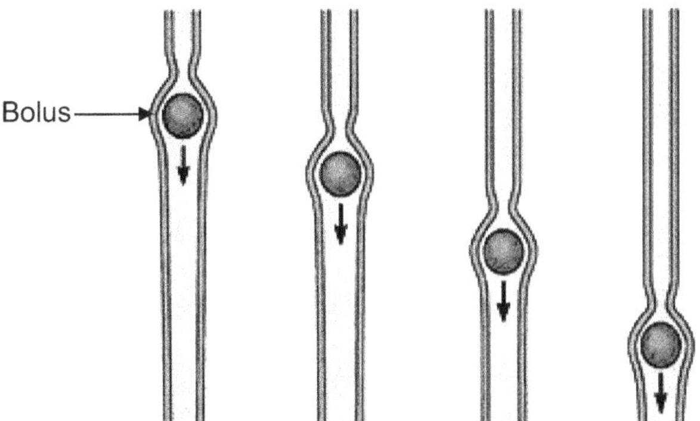

Fig. 2.17: Peristalsis in small intestine

2.18 CHEMICAL DIGESTION IN SMALL INTESTINE

Digestion of carbohydrates:

- Pancreatic amylase converts all polysaccharides into monosaccarides.
- α-dextrinase a brush-border enzyme converts starch into smaller fragments.
- Sucrase enzyme breaks sucrose into a molecule of glucose and a molecule of fructose
- Lactase enzyme digests lactose into a molecule of glucose and a molecule of galactose
- Maltase enzyme splits maltose and maltotriose into two or three molecules of glucose, respectively.

Digestion of proteins:

- Enzymes in pancreatic juice-trypsin, chymotrypsin and carboxypeptidase convert all proteins to amino acids.

Digestion of fats:

- The enzyme lingual lipase, gastric lipase and pancreatic lipase converts fats to fatty acid and glycerol.

Digestion of nucleic acids:

- Pancreatic juice contains two types of nucleases, ribonuclease, which digests RNA, and deoxyribonuclease, which digests DNA.
- The nucleotides that result from the action of two nucleases are further digested by brush-border enzymes called nucleosidases and phosphatases into pentoses, phosphates and nitrogenous bases.

2.19 ABSORPTION IN THE SMALL INTESTINE

- All the chemical and mechanical phases of digestion from the mouth through the small intestine are directed toward changing food into forms that can pass through the absorptive epithelial cells lining the mucosa and into the underlying blood and lymphatic vessels.
- These forms are monosaccharides (glucose, fructose and galactose) from carbohydrates; single amino acids, dipeptides and tripeptides from proteins; and fatty acids, glycerol, and monoglycerides from triglycerides.

- Passage of these digested nutrients from the gastrointestinal tract into the blood or lymph is called absorption.
- Absorption of materials occurs via diffusion, facilitated diffusion, osmosis and active transport.
- About 90% of all absorption of nutrients occurs in the small intestine; the other 10% occurs in the stomach and large intestine.
- Any undigested or unabsorbed material left in the small intestine passes on to the large intestine.

Absorption of Monosaccharides:

- All carbohydrates are absorbed as monosaccharides.
- The capacity of small intestine to absorb monosaccharides is huge 120 grams per hour.
- Monosaccharides pass from the lumen through the apical membrane via facilitated diffusion or active transport.
- Fructose, a monosaccharide found in fruits, is transported via facilitated diffusion.
- Glucose and galactose are transported into absorptive cells of villi via secondary active transport with Na^+.

Absorption of Amino Acids, Dipeptides and Tripeptides:

- Most proteins are absorbed as amino acids via active transport processes that occur mainly in duodenum and jejunum.
- Some amino acids enter absorptive cells of the villi via Na^+ dependent secondary active transport processes and other amino acids are actively transported.
- Dipeptides and Tripeptides are transported by secondary active transport with H^+.

Absorption of Lipids:

- All dietary lipids are absorbed via simple diffusion process.
- As a result of digestion the triglycerides are broken down into monoglycerides and fatty acids, which can be either short-chain fatty acid or long-chain fatty acids.
- Although short-chain fatty acids are hydrophobic, they are very small in size.
- Because of their small size, they can dissolve in the watery intestinal chyme, pass through the absorptive cells via simple diffusion.
- Long-chain fatty acids and monoglycerides are large and hydrophobic and have difficulty being suspended in the watery environment of the intestinal chyme they forms micelle and undergoes transportation by simple diffusion process.
- Once formed, the micelles move from the interior of small intestinal lumen to the brush border of absorptive cells.
- At that point, the long-chain fatty acids and monoglycerides diffuse out of the micelles into the absorptive cells, leaving the micelles behind in the chyme.
- Once inside the absorptive cells, long-chain fatty acids and monoglycerides are recombined to form triglycerides, which aggregate into globules along with phospholipids, cholesterol and become coated with proteins.

- These large spherical masses are called chylomicrons (80 mm in diameter).
- Chylomicrons leave the absorptive cell via exocytosis because of large size and bulkiness chylomicrons cannot enter the blood capillaries (pores in the walls of blood capillaries are too small).
- Instead of that chylomicrons enter lacteals that have much larger pores than blood capillaries.
- From lacteals, chylomicrons are transported via lymphatic vessels to the blood circulation.

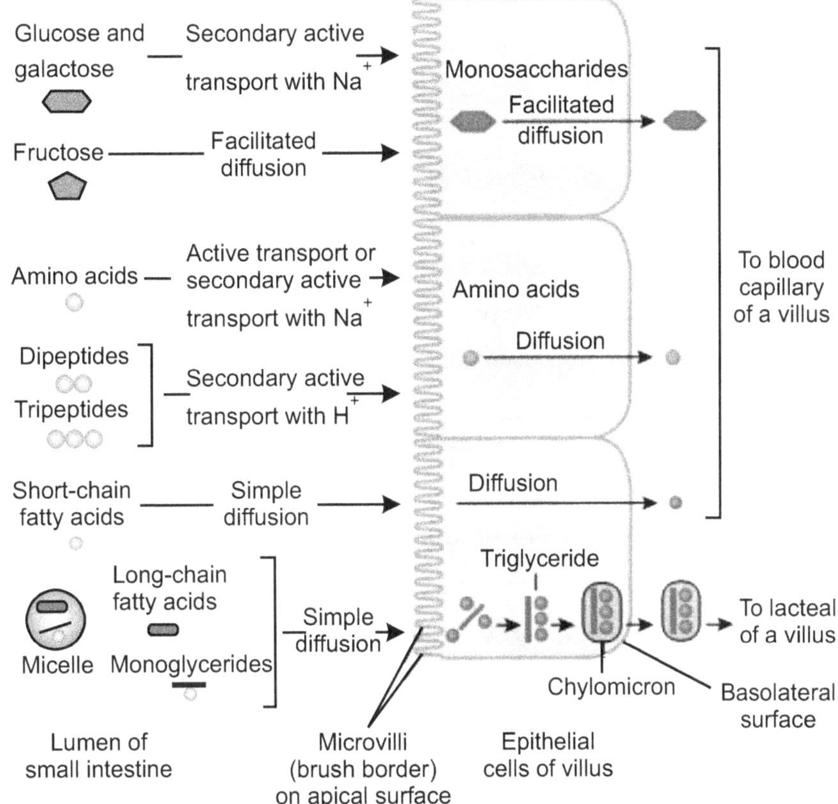

Fig. 2.18: Movement of nutrients through absorptive epithelial cells of villi

2.20 PANCREAS

- It is yellowish in colour and elongated leaf shaped gland lying behind the stomach.
- It is about 12-15 cm long and 2.5 cm thick.
- It consists of three parts. Head, Body and Tail
- The head is expanded portion and lies near the curve of the duodenum.
- To the left of head are the central body and the tapering tail.
- Pancreas is functionally divided into two parts.
  - ✓ **Exocrine pancreas:** It is made up of small clusters of glandular epithelium cells, about 99% of which are arranged in clusters called as acini and constitute exocrine

portion of organ. The cells within the acini secrete a mixture of fluid and digestive enzymes called as pancreatic juice.

✓ **Endocrine pancreas:** Remaining 1% of cells are arranged into clusters called as pancreatic islets (islets of Langerhans). The cells secrete the hormone insulin, glucagon which is responsible for maintenance of blood sugar level. Insulin lowers the blood sugar level whereas; glucagon increases the blood sugar level.

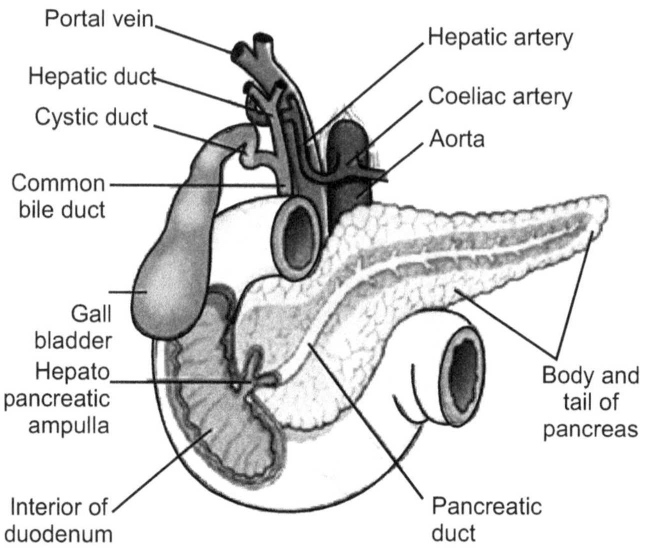

Fig. 2.19: Pancreas and associated structure

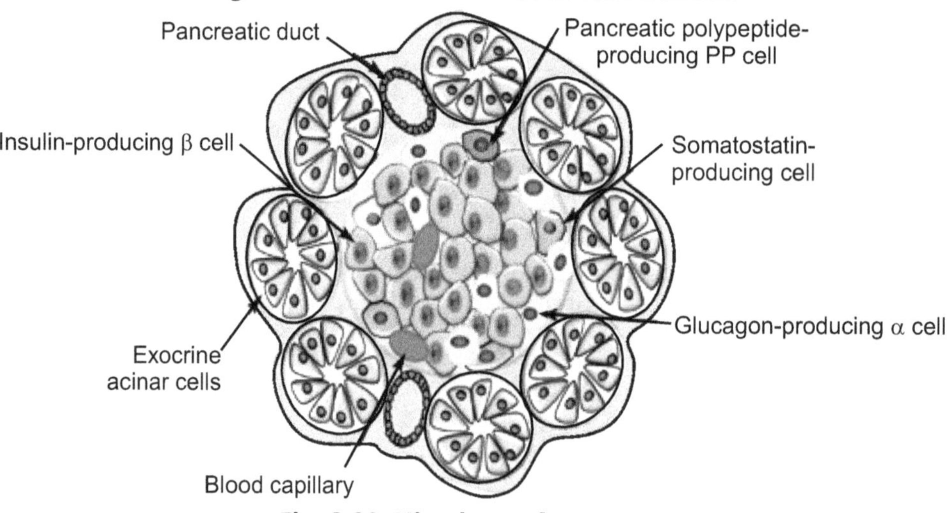

Fig. 2.20: Histology of pancreas

2.21 PANCREATIC JUICE

- It is clear, colourless liquid consists of water, salts, sodium bicarbonate (alkaline pH 7.1-8.2) and several enzymes.

- Each day pancreas produces 1.2 to 1.5 liter of pancreatic juice.
- The enzyme in pancreatic juice includes:
  - **Carbohydrate digesting enzyme:** Pancreatin amylase
  - **Protein digesting enzyme:** Trypsin, Chymotrypsin, Carboxypeptidase and Elastase
  - **Triglyceride digesting enzyme:** Pancreatic lipase
  - **Nucleic acid digesting enzyme:** Ribonuclease and Deoxyribonuclease

Functions

- It neutralizes acidic contents of chyme in the duodenum due to the presence of high bicarbonate solution.
- Pancreatic juice provides alkaline pH for enzyme action.
- Glycogen, starch and other complex carbohydrate are hydrolyzed to disaccharides by pancreatic α-amylase.
- Enzyme nucleotides digest nucleoproteins.
- Proteins are converted to amino acid by enzyme pancreatic trypsin, chymotrypsin and elastase.
- Pancreatic lipase hydrolyses fats to fatty acid and glycerol.

2.22 LIVER

- It is a largest gland of the body, weighing about 1.4 kg in an average adult.
- It is situated in the upper part of abdominal cavity.
- Externally, liver is covered with peritoneum.
- It is divided into two principal lobes i.e. right lobe and left lobe by falciform ligaments (a fold of the peritoneum).
- Right lobe is again divided into;
  - ✓ Caudate lobe
  - ✓ Quadrate lobe
- The lobes of liver are made up of many functional units called as lobules.
- Lobule is typically six-sided structure (hexagon) that consists of specialized epithelial cells called as hepatocytes arranged in irregular, branching, interconnected plates around the central vein.
- Liver lobules contain highly permeable capillaries called as sinusoids, through which blood passes.
- In sinusoids fixed phagocytes are present called as stellate reticuloendothelial (Kupffer) cells, which destroy worn out WBC, RBC, bacteria and foreign matter in the blood.
- The hepatocytes secrete bile into small intracellular canals called as bile canaliculi.
- These bile canaliculi pass bile into bile ducts.
- The bile ducts merge and form the larger right and left hepatic ducts which unite and exit the liver as the common hepatic duct.

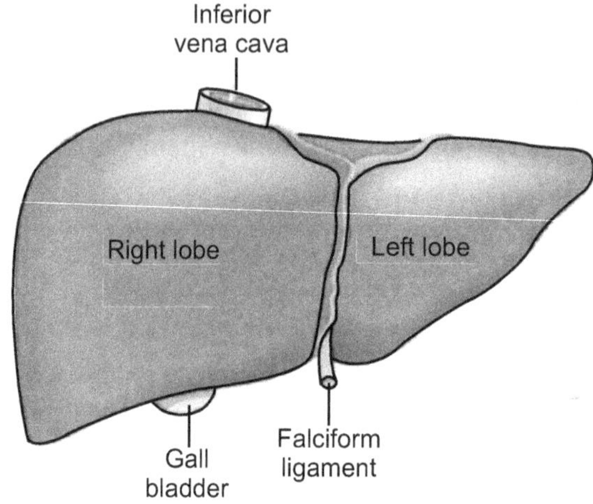

Fig. 2.21: Liver

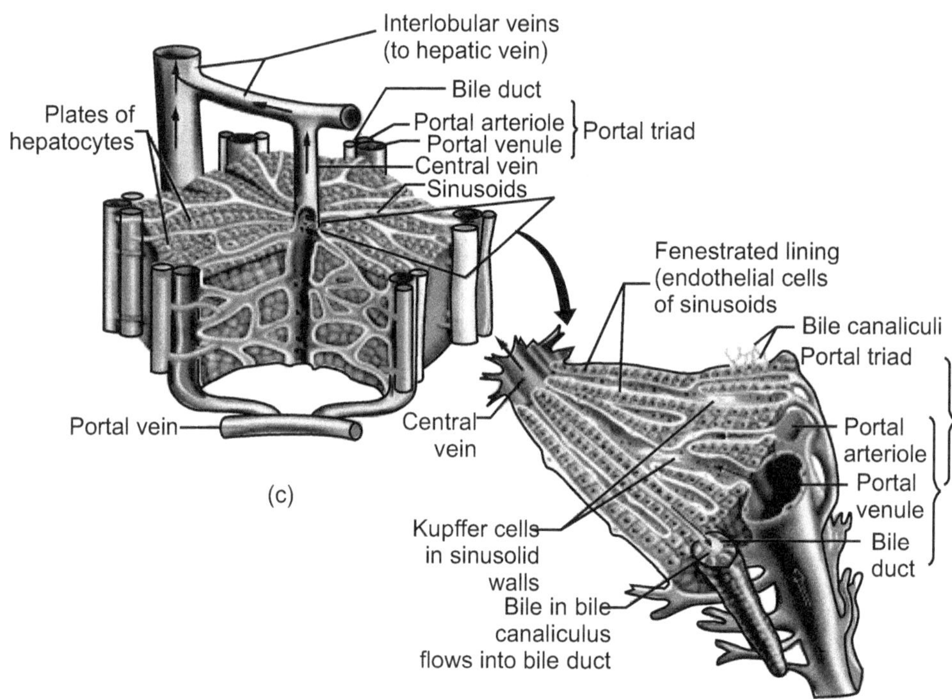

Fig. 2.22: Hepatocyte

Blood supply to liver: It receives blood from two sources.

✓ **Hepatic artery:** It obtains oxygenated blood.

✓ **Hepatic vein:** It receives deoxygenated blood containing newly absorbed nutrients, drug and microbes, toxins from GI tract.

Functions of liver

Functions related to metabolism

(a) Carbohydrate metabolism
- ✓ Liver stores glycogen.
- ✓ Liver converts fructose and galactose to glucose.
- ✓ Liver causes gluconeogenesis.
- ✓ Liver leads to glycogenolysis i.e. breakdown of glycogen and glucose.

(b) Fat metabolism
- ✓ Liver produces energy through oxidation of fatty acids.
- ✓ It leads to formation of lipoproteins.
- ✓ It synthesizes large amount of cholesterol and phospholipids.
- ✓ It converts large number of carbohydrates and proteins into fat.

(c) Protein metabolism
- ✓ Liver causes deamination of amino acid.
- ✓ It removes ammonia from the body by converting it into urea.
- ✓ Parenchymal cells of liver synthesize albumin and plasma proteins.

Activation of vitamin-D
- The skin, liver and kidneys participate in synthesizing the active form of vitamin-D.

Excretion of bilirubin
- Bilirubin derived from the heme of aged RBC's is absorbed by the liver from blood and secreted into bile. Most of the bilirubin in bile is metabolized in the small intestine by bacteria and eliminated in faeces.

Storage
- The liver is a prime storage site for certain vitamin (A, B_{12}, D, E and K) and minerals (iron and copper).

Breakdown of RBC's and defense against microbes
- This is carried out by phagocytic hepatic macrophages (Kupffer cells) in the sinusoids.

Detoxification of drugs and noxious substances
- This includes ethanol (alcohol) and toxins produced by microbes.

Production of heat
- Liver is a major heat producing organ of body.

2.23 GALL BLADDER

- It is a pear shaped sac attached to posterior surface of the liver.
- It is 7-10 cm long.
- It has fundus (expanded end), a body (main part) and neck that are continuous with the cystic duct.
- When food enters the small intestine, a hormone called as cholecystokinin is released.
- Cholecystokinin signals the gall bladder to contract and secrete bile into the small intestine through the common bile duct.

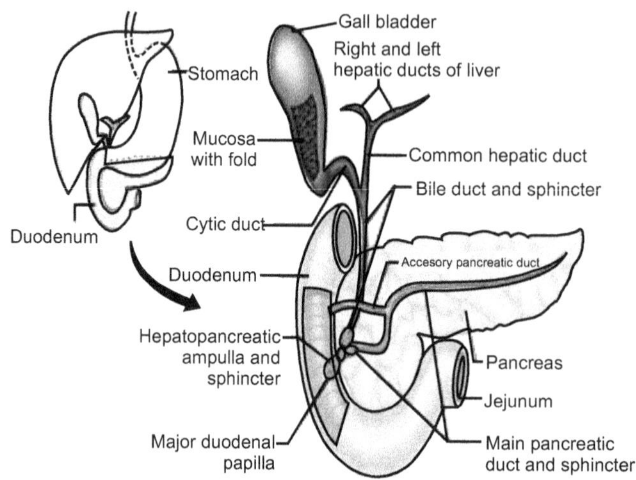

Fig. 2.23: Gall bladder and associated structure

Function

- Its store and concentrate bile.
- It acts as a reservoir for bile.
- It releases stored bile.

2.24 BILE

- It is secreted by the liver; therefore it passes from the hepatic duct along the cystic duct to the gall bladder where it is stored.
- Near about 500-1000 ml of bile is secreted daily.
- It has alkaline pH 8.
- It consists of:
  - ✓ Water
  - ✓ Mineral salts
  - ✓ Mucus
  - ✓ Bile salt
  - ✓ Bile pigments (Bilirubin)
  - ✓ Cholesterol

Functions

- The bile salts emulsify fats in the small intestine.
- Fatty acids are insoluble in water which makes them difficult to absorb through the intestinal wall.
- Bile salts make cholesterol and fatty acid soluble.

2.25 LARGE INTESTINE (LI)

- It is the terminal portion of gastro-intestinal tract.
- It is about 1.5 m long and 6.5 cm in diameter extends from the ileum to the anus.
- It forms arch around the coiled small intestine.

- The colon is divided into the,
  - ✓ Caecum
  - ✓ Ascending colon
  - ✓ Transverse colon
  - ✓ Descending colon
  - ✓ Sigmoid colon
  - ✓ Rectum
  - ✓ Anal canal

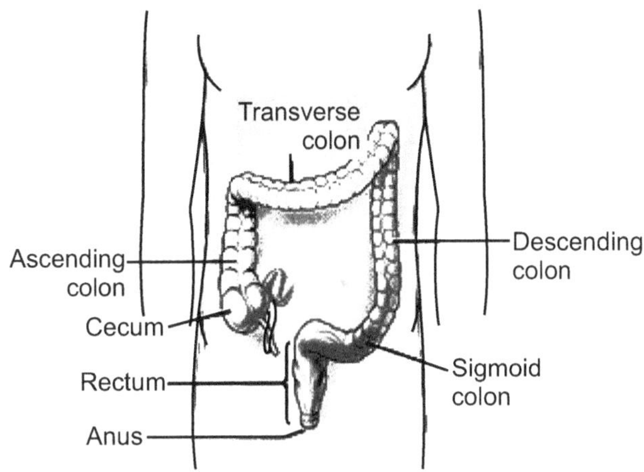

Fig. 2.24: Large intestine

Caecum

- It is first part of the colon.
- The elevated portion of large intestine below the ileocaecal sphincter is caecum.
- To the caecum a twisted coiled tube is attached called as appendix or vermiform appendix.

Colon

- The remaining part of the large intestine is called as colon.
- The colon is divided into four basic parts.
  - ✓ **Ascending colon**: It ascends on the right side of the abdomen, reaches the inferior surface of the liver and turns abruptly to the left to form the right colic (hepatic) flexure.
  - ✓ **Transverse colon**: It curves beneath the inferior end of the spleen on the left side as the left colic (splenic) flexure.
  - ✓ **Descending colon**: It passes inferiorly to the level of iliac crest.
  - ✓ **Sigmoid colon**: It begins near the left iliac crest, projects medially to the midline and terminates as the rectum.

Rectum

- It is a dilated section of the colon of about 13 cm long.
- It leads from the sigmoid colon and terminates in the anal canal.

- It stores faeces which consist of undigested part of food, water, inorganic salts and bacteria, etc.

Anal canal

- This is a short passage about 3.8 cm long that leads from the rectum to the exterior.
- The mucous membrane of the anal canal is arranged in longitudinal folds called anal columns that contain a network of arteries and veins.
- The opening of anal canal to the exterior, called as anus, is guarded by an internal anal sphincter of smooth muscle and an external anal sphincter of skeletal muscle.
- These sphincters keep the anus closed except during the elimination of faeces.

Functions

Absorption

- In large intestine absorption of water by osmosis, continues until the semisolid consistency of faeces is achieved.
- Mineral salts, vitamins and some drugs are also absorbed into the blood capillaries from the large intestine.

Microbial activity

- The large intestine is heavily colonized by certain types of bacteria which synthesize certain vitamins and folic acid i.e. *E. coli, S. faecalis.*
- These microbes are the normal flora of the large intestine in human.
- However, they may become pathogenic if transferred to another part of the body e.g. *E. coli* may cause cystitis if it gains access to the urinary bladder.

Defecation reflex

- Mass peristalsis movements push fecal material from the sigmoid colon into the rectum.
- The resulting distension of the rectal wall stimulates stretch receptors which initiates a defecation reflex that empties the rectum.

2.26 DISORDERS OF DIGESTIVE SYSTEM

Dental caries/Tooth decay

- It involves a gradual demineralization (softening) of the enamel and dentin.
- If untreated micro-organism may invade the pulp causing inflammation and infection with subsequent death of the pulp and abscess of the alveolar bone surrounding the root apex requiring root canal therapy.

Periodontal disease

- It is a collective term for a variety of conditions characterized by inflammation and degeneration of the gingivae, alveolar bone, periodontal ligament and cement.
- These diseases are often caused by poor oral hygiene, by local irritants such as bacteria, impacted food and cigarette smoke.

Peptic ulcer diseases (PUD)

- An ulcer is a craterlike lesion in a membrane.
- Ulcers that develop in the areas of gastrointestinal tract exposed to the acidic gastric juice are called as peptic ulcer.

- The most common complications of peptic ulcer is bleeding which can lead to anemia if enough blood is lost.
- The causes of PUD are
  - ✓ Bacteria - *Helicobacter pylori*
  - ✓ Non-steroidal anti-inflammatory drugs
  - ✓ Hypersecretions of HCl

Diverticular diseases

- In diverticular disease, saclike out pouching of the wall of colon occurs termed as diverticula.
- The development of diverticula is called as diverticulosis.
- Diverticula showing inflammation is called as diverticulitis.
- The condition may be characterized by pain either constipation or increased frequency of defecation, nausea, vomiting and low grade fever.

Colorectal cancer

- The cancer of colon and rectum is called as colorectal cancer.
- Intake of alcohol and diet high in proteins and fats are associated with increased risk of colorectal cancer.

Hepatitis

- It is an inflammation of the liver that can be caused by viruses, drugs and chemicals including alcohol.
- Types of hepatitis:
  - ✓ **Hepatitis-A:** It is caused by the hepatitis A virus and is spread via fecal contamination of objects such as food, clothing, toys and eating utensils (fecal–oral route).
  - ✓ **Hepatitis-B:** It is caused by the hepatitis B virus and is spread primarily by sexual contact, contaminated syringes and transfusion equipment. It can also be spread via saliva and tears.
  - ✓ **Hepatitis-C:** It is caused by the hepatitis C virus, is clinically similar to hepatitis B.
  - ✓ **Hepatitis-D:** It is caused by the hepatitis D virus. It is transmitted like hepatitis B and in fact a person must have been co-infected with hepatitis B before contracting hepatitis D.
  - ✓ **Hepatitis-E:** It is caused by the hepatitis E virus and is spread like hepatitis A.

Anorexia nervosa

- It is chronic disorder characterised by self-induced weight loss, negative perception of body image and physiological changes that results from nutritional depletion.
- Patients of anorexia nervosa have a fixation on weight control and often insist on having a bowel movement every day despite inadequate food intake.

QUESTIONS

Short Answer Questions

1. Define digestion and gastroenterology.
2. Draw a labeled diagram of digestive system.
3. Write a note on small and large intestine.
4. Write a note on function of pancreas.
5. Describe the structure and functions of salivary glands.
6. Write a note on gastric juice and its functions.
7. Write a note on role of enzymes in digestion.
8. Enlist organs involved in digestive system and give function of each organ.
9. Enlist and define disorders of pancreatic islets.
10. Explain the structure and function of liver.
11. Draw a neat labeled diagram of digestive system and explain functions of liver.
12. Explain structure and functions of stomach.
13. Explain the process of digestion in the stomach.

Long Answer Questions:

1. Give the anatomy and physiology of different parts of digestive system along with neat labeled diagram.
2. Explain the process of absorption, chemical and mechanical digestion in small intestine.

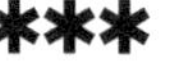

UNIT III

Chapter **3**...

ENERGETICS

◆ LEARNING OBJECTIVES ◆

❖ To study the structure of Adenosine triphosphate.

❖ To describe the process of formation of ATP by cellular respiration.

❖ To describe the process of anaerobic and aerobic cellular respiration.

❖ To study the concept of basal metabolic rate and factors affecting on basal metabolic rate.

3.1 INTRODUCTION

The food material we are eating is the only source of energy for walking, running, breathing and performing other body activities. Carbohydrates, lipid and proteins material present in the food is digested by various enzymes and absorbed in the gastrointestinal tract. After digestion the products of digestion such as; monosaccarides, fatty acids, glycerides, amino acids, minerals and vitamins reaches the body cells. The food molecules absorbed by the gastrointestinal tract have three important applications such as;

- Most of the food molecules are used to supply energy for sustaining life processes such as DNA replication, protein synthesis, muscle contraction, maintenance of body temperature and mitosis.

- Some food molecules are used for the building blocks of complex molecules such as muscle proteins, hormones and enzymes.

- Other food molecules are stored for future use such as glycogen in liver cells and triglycerides in adipose cells.

3.2 Metabolic Reactions

Metabolism

- It is a term used to describe all the chemical reactions involved in maintaining the living state of the cells and the organism.

- It is an energy-balancing act between catabolic (decomposition) reactions and anabolic (synthesis) reactions.

- There are two types of metabolism reactions:
  - ✓ Catabolism: Breakdown of molecules to obtain energy.
  - ✓ Anabolism: Synthesis of all molecules needed by the cells.

(3.1)

Catabolism

- These chemical reactions involve the breakdown of complex organic molecules into simpler ones.
- Catabolic (decomposition) reactions are exergonic means they produce more energy than they consume and releasing the chemical energy stored in organic molecules.
- Examples of catabolic reactions are:
  - ✓ Glycolysis
  - ✓ Krebs cycle
  - ✓ Electron transport chain

Anabolism

- These chemical reactions involve combining of simple molecules to form the body's complex structural and functional components.
- Anabolic (synthesis) reactions are endergonic means they consume more energy than they produce.
- Examples of anabolic reactions are the formation of peptide bonds between amino acids during protein synthesis, the building of fatty acids into phospholipids that form the plasma membrane bilayer and the linkage of glucose monomers to form glycogen.

3.3 ADENOSINE TRIPHOSPHATE (ATP)

- ATP molecule participates in most of energy exchange reaction in living cells that combines catabolic reactions to anabolic reactions.
- The metabolic reactions depends on the activeness of enzymes in a particular cell at a particular time.
- Catabolic reactions occur in the mitochondria and at the same time anabolic reactions occur in the endoplasmic reticulum of a cell.
- ATP is called as "energy currency" of a living cell.
- A typical cell has about a billion of ATP molecules, each being lasts for less than a minute before being used.
- Thus, it is not long term source of energy.
- A molecule of ATP consists of an adenine molecule, a ribose molecule, and three phosphate groups bonded to one another.

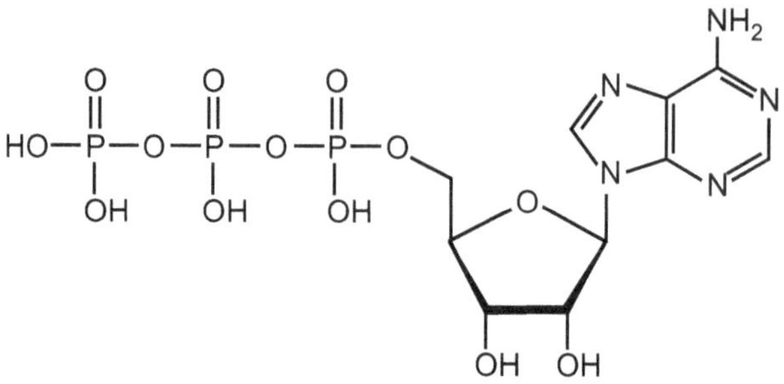

Fig. 3.1: Structure of Adenosine Triphosphate

- When the terminal phosphate group is removed from ATP, adenosine diphosphate (ADP) and a phosphate group (P) are formed.
- Some of the energy get released during this process is used to drive anabolic reactions such as the formation of glycogen from glucose.
- In addition to that, energy from various complex molecules is used in catabolic reactions to combine ADP and a phosphate group to from ATP.

$$ADP + P + Energy \longrightarrow ATP$$

- Nearby 40% of the energy released in catabolism reaction is used for cellular functions and remaining amount is converted to heat that helps in maintaining normal body temperature. Excess heat is lost to the environment.

3.3.1 Formation of ATP by Cellular Respiration

- The oxidation of glucose to produce ATP is known as cellular respiration.
- Cellular respiration involves four sets of reactions:
  - ✓ Glycolysis
  - ✓ Formation of acetyl coenzyme-A
  - ✓ Krebs cycle
  - ✓ Electron transport chain

Glycolysis:

- It is a set of reactions in which one glucose molecule is oxidized and two molecules of pyruvic acid are produced.
- The reactions also produce two molecules of ATP and two energy-containing NADH, H^+.
- Because glycolysis does not require oxygen, it is a way to produce ATP anaerobically (without oxygen) and is known as anaerobic cellular respiration.
- During glycolysis, chemical reactions split a 6-carbon molecule of glucose into two 3-carbon molecules of pyruvic acid.
- Even though glycolysis consumes two ATP molecules, it produces four ATP molecules, for a net gain of two ATP molecules for each glucose.

Formation of acetyl coenzyme A:

- It is a transition step that prepares pyruvic acid for entrance into the Krebs cycle.
- This step also produces energy-containing NADH, H^+ and carbon dioxide (CO_2).

Krebs cycle reactions:

- It oxidizes acetyl coenzyme A and produce CO_2, ATP, energy-containing NADH, H^+ and $FADH_2$.

Electron transport chain reactions:

- It oxidizes NADH, H^+ and $FADH_2$ and transfers their electrons through a series of electron carriers.
- The Krebs cycle and the electron transport chain both require oxygen to produce ATP and are collectively known as aerobic cellular respiration.

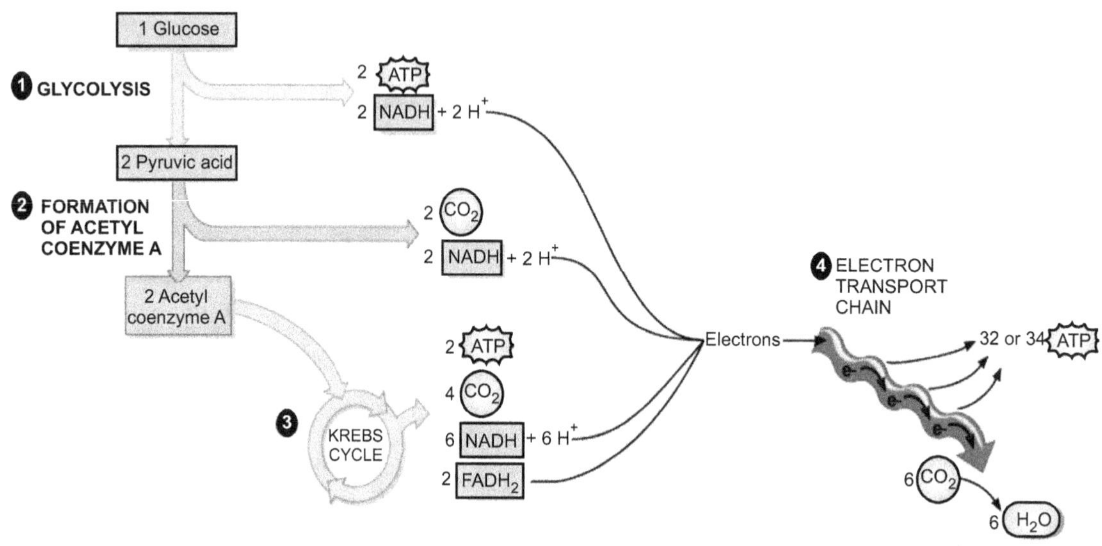

Fig. 3.2: Cellular respiration

Muscle metabolism:

- For muscle contraction, ATP must be available in the muscle fiber.
- ATP is available from the following sources:
- ATP available within the muscle fiber can maintain muscle contraction for several seconds.
- Creatine phosphate, a high- energy molecule stored in muscle cells, transfers its high energy phosphate group to ADP to form ATP. The creatine phosphate in muscle cells is able to generate enough ATP to maintain muscle contraction for about 15 seconds.
- Glucose within the cell is stored in the carbohydrate glycogen. Through the metabolic process of glycogenolysis, glycogen is broken down to release glucose. ATP is then generated from glucose by cellular respiration.
- When energy requirements are high, glucose from glycogen stored in the liver and fatty acids from fat stored in adipose cells and the liver are released into the bloodstream. Glucose and fatty acids are then absorbed from the bloodstream by muscle cells. ATP is then generated from these energy rich molecules by cellular respiration.

Production of ATP in muscle fibers:

- Muscle fibers have three ways to produce ATP.
- From creatine phosphate
- By anaerobic cellular respiration
- By aerobic cellular respiration
- The use of creatine phosphate for ATP production is unique to muscle fibers, but all body cells make ATP by the reactions of anaerobic and aerobic cellular respiration.

Creatine Phosphate:

- When muscle fibers are relaxed, they produce more ATP than they need for resting metabolism.
- The excess ATP is used to synthesize creatine phosphate, an energy-rich molecule that is found only in muscle fibers.
- The enzyme creatine kinase (CK) catalyzes the transfer of high-energy phosphate groups from ATP to creatine, forming creatine phosphate and ADP.
- Creatine is a small, amino acid like molecule that is synthesized in the liver, kidneys, pancreas and then transported to muscle fibers.
- Creatine phosphate is three to six times more plentiful than ATP in the sarcoplasm of a relaxed muscle fiber.
- When contraction begins and the ADP level starts to rise, CK catalyzes the transfer of a high-energy phosphate group from creatine phosphate back to ADP.
- This direct phosphorylation reaction quickly regenerates new ATP molecules.
- Together, creatine phosphate and ATP provide enough energy for muscles to contract maximally for about 15 seconds.

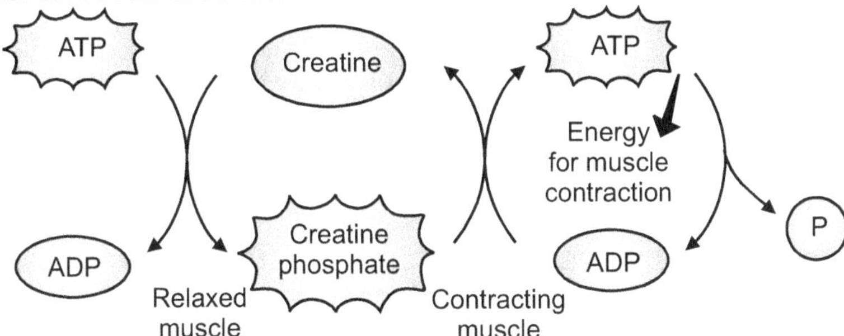

Fig. 3.3: Production of ATP by creatine phosphate

Anaerobic cellular respiration:

- It is a series of ATP-producing reactions that do not require oxygen.
- When muscle activity continues and the supply of creatine phosphate within the muscle fiber is depleted, glucose is catabolized to generate ATP.
- Glucose easily passes from the blood into contracting muscle fibers via facilitated diffusion, and it is also produced by the breakdown of glycogen within muscle fibers.
- Then, a series of 10 reactions known as glycolysis quickly breaks down each glucose molecule into two molecules of pyruvic acid.
- These reactions use two molecules of ATP but produce four molecules of ATP.
- Thus, there is net gain of two molecules of ATP.
- Anaerobic reactions convert most of the pyruvic acid to lactic acid in the cytosol.
- Anaerobic cellular respiration can provide enough energy for about 30 to 40 seconds of maximal muscle activity.

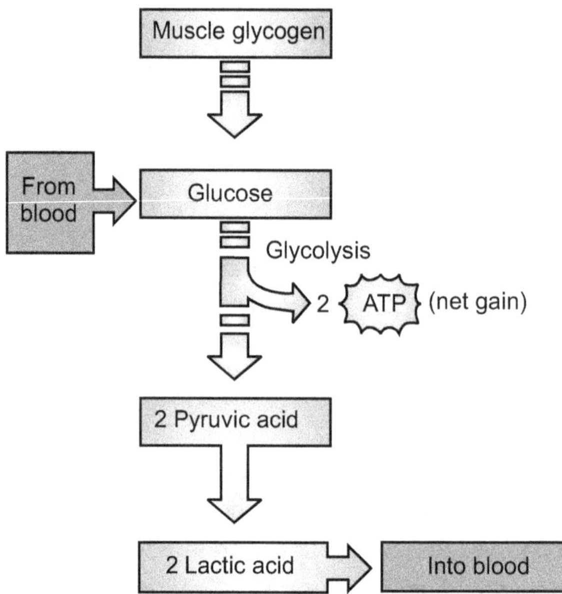

Fig. 3.4: Production of ATP by anaerobic cellular respiration

Aerobic Cellular Respiration:

- It is series of oxygen-requiring reactions that produce ATP in mitochondria.
- The pyruvic acid formed by glycolysis in the cytosol enters the mitochondria, where it undergoes a series of oxygen-requiring reactions called as aerobic cellular respiration that produce a large amount of ATP.
- If sufficient oxygen is present, pyruvic acid enters the mitochondria, where it is completely oxidized in reactions that generate ATP, carbon dioxide, water and heat.
- Aerobic cellular respiration is slower than glycolysis, it yields much more ATP.
- Each molecule of glucose yields about 36 molecules of ATP; a typical fatty acid molecule yields more than 100 molecules of ATP via aerobic cellular respiration.

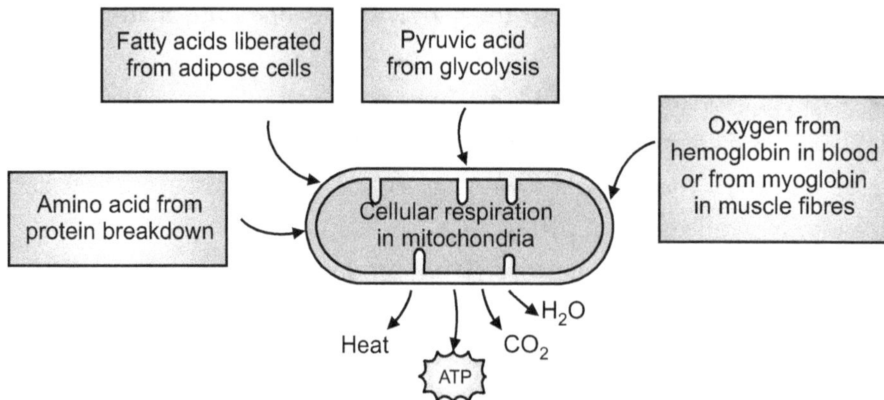

Fig. 3.5: Production of ATP by aerobic cellular respiration

3.4 BASAL METABOLIC RATE (BMR)

- It is the energy released when the subject is at complete mental and physical rest i.e. in a room with comfortable temperature and humidity, awake and sitting in a reclining position, 10-12 hours after the last meal.
- It is essentially the minimum energy required to maintain the heart rate, respiration, kidney function etc.
- The BMR of an average adult is 1200-1800 Kcal/day.

Factors Influencing BMR:
- There are many factors that affect the BMR.
- These include body temperature, age, sex, race, emotional state, climate and circulating levels of hormones like catecholamine's (epinephrine and norepinephrine) and those secreted by the thyroid gland.

Genetics (Race):
- Some people are born with faster metabolism and some with slower metabolism.
- Indians and Chinese seem to have a lower BMR than the Europeans.
- This may occurs due to dietary differences between these races.
- Higher BMR exists in individuals living in tropical climates. e.g. Singapore.

Age:
- BMR reduces with age i.e. it is inversely proportional to age.
- Children have higher BMR than adults.

Gender:
- Men have a greater muscle mass and a lower body fat percentage.
- Thus men have a higher basal metabolic rate than women.
- The BMR of females declines more rapidly between the ages of 5 and 17 than that of males.

Weight:
- The heavier the weight, the higher the BMR, e.g. the metabolic rate of obese women is 25 percent higher than that of thin women.

Body surface area:
- This is a reflection of the height and weight.
- The greater the body surface area factor, the higher the BMR.
- Tall, thin people have higher BMRs.

Diet:
- Starvation or serious abrupt calorie-reduction can dramatically reduce BMR by up to 30%.
- Restrictive low-calorie weight loss diets may cause BMR to drop as much as 20%.
- BMR of strict vegetarians is 11% lower than that of meat eaters.

Body fat percentage:
- The lower the body fat percentage, the higher the BMR.
- The lower body fat percentage in the male body is one reason why men generally have a 10-15% higher BMR than women.

Body temperature/health:
- For every increase of 0.5°C in internal temperature of the body, the BMR increases by about 7 percent.
- The chemical reactions in the body actually occur more quickly at higher temperatures.
- So a patient with a fever of 42° C would have an increase of about 50 percent in BMR.
- An increase in body temperature as a result of fever increases the BMR by 14-15% per degree centigrade which evidently, is due to the increased rate of metabolic reactions of the body.

External temperature:
- Temperature outside the body also affects basal metabolic rate.
- Exposure to cold temperature causes an increase in the BMR, so as to create the extra heat needed to maintain the body's internal temperature.
- A short exposure to hot temperature has little effect on the body's metabolism as it is compensated mainly by increased heat loss.
- But prolonged exposure to heat can raise BMR.

Glands:
- Thyroxine is a key BMR-regulator which speeds up the metabolic activity of the body.
- The more thyroxine produced, the higher the BMR. If too much thyroxine is produced (thyrotoxicosis) BMR can actually double. If too little thyroxine is produced (myxoedema) BMR may shrink to 30-40 percent of normal rate.

Exercise:
- Physical exercise not only influences body weight by burning calories, it also helps raise the BMR by building extra lean tissue.
- So more calories are burnt even when sleeping.

Pregnancy:
- The BMR is not changed during pregnancy.
- The higher value of BMR in late pregnancy is due to the BMR of the foetus.

Significance of BMR:
- The determination of BMR is the guide for diagnosis and treatment of thyroid disorders.
- If BMR is less than 10% of the normal, it indicates moderate hypothyroidism. In severe hypothyroidism, the BMR may be decreased to 40 to 50 percent below normal.
- The BMR is low in starvation, under nutrition, hypothalamic disorders, Addison's disease and lipoid nephrosis.
- BMR aids to know the total amount of food or calories required to maintain body weight.
- The BMR is above normal in fever, diabetes insipidus, leukemia and polycythemia.

QUESTIONS

Short Answer Questions:
1. What is ATP?
2. Describe the process of formation of ATP.
3. Explain the process of anaerobic respiration.
4. What is BMR?
5. Enlist the factors affecting on BMR.

UNIT III

Chapter **4**...

RESPIRATORY SYSTEM

♦ LEARNING OBJECTIVES ♦

❖ To describe the anatomy and physiology of the nose, pharynx, larynx, trachea, bronchi, and lungs.

❖ To study the physiology of voice production.

❖ To describe the mechanism of external and internal respiration.

❖ To study the transports of oxygen and carbon dioxide.

❖ To study different lung volume and capacities.

❖ To describe methods of artificial respiration.

4.1 INTRODUCTION

The respiratory system is a biological system consisting of specific organs and structures used for the respiration process in an organism. It is involved in the intake and exchange of oxygen and carbon dioxide between an organism and the environment.

The branch of medicine that deals with the diagnosis and treatment of diseases of ears, nose and throat is called as Otorhinolaryngology.

4.2 RESPIRATION

- The oxidative process occurring within living cells by which the chemical energy of organic molecules is released in a series of metabolic steps involving the consumption of oxygen and the liberation of carbon dioxide and water is called as respiration.

- The process of respiration is divided into 3 different processes
  - ✓ **Pulmonary ventilation:** It is the inspiration (inflow) and expiration (outflow) of air between the atmosphere and the lungs.
  - ✓ **External respiration:** It is the exchange of gases between the lungs and the blood.
  - ✓ **Internal respiration**: It is the exchange of gases between the blood and the body cells.

(4.1)

4.3 CLASSIFICATION OF RESPIRATORY SYSTEM

- Anatomically it is divided into:

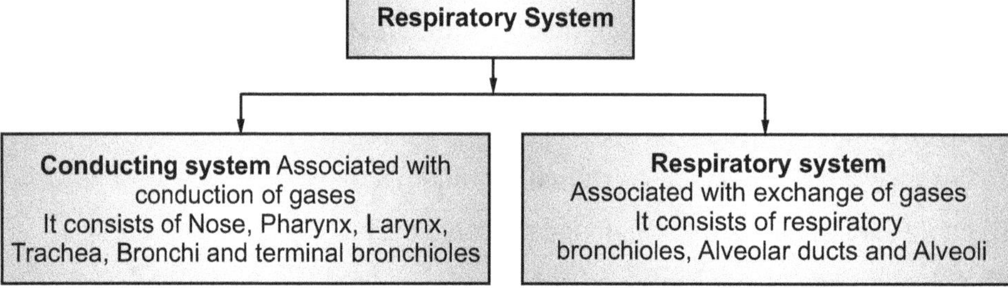

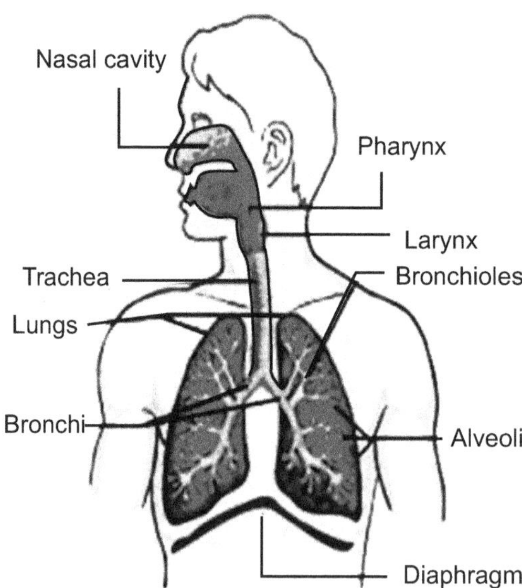

Fig. 4.1: Respiratory system

4.4 UPPER RESPIRATORY SYSTEM

NOSE

- It is a structure of the face made of cartilage, bone, muscle and skin that supports and protects the anterior portion of the nasal cavity.
- It is the external portion of respiratory system and open through the nostrils.

- The nasal cavity is divided by a septum into left and right portion.
- The nasal cavity is a hollow space within the nose that is lined with hair and mucus membrane.
- The nose is lined by vascular ciliated columnar epithelium containing mucus secreting goblet cells.

Functions

- It warms, moisturise and filter the air entering the body before it reaches the lungs.
- Hair and mucus lining of the nasal cavity helps to trap dust, mold, pollen and other environmental contaminants before they can reach the inner portions of body.
- Air exiting the body through the nose returns moisture and heat to the nasal cavity before being exhaled into the environment.
- It is the organ of sense of smell. The nerve endings that detect the smell are located in the roof of nose.

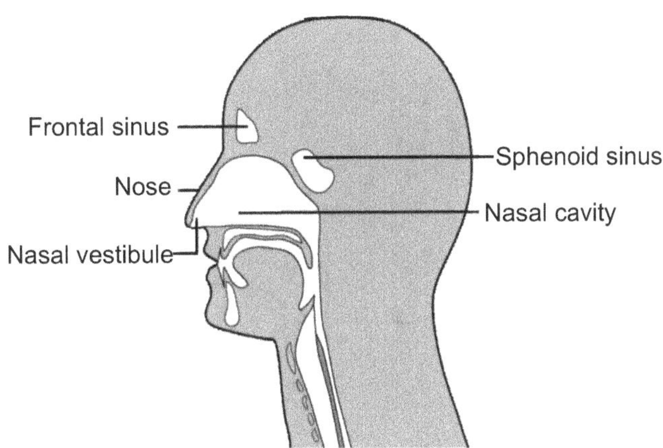

Fig. 4.2: Nose

4.5 PHARYNX

- The pharynx or throat is a funnel shaped tube of about 13 cm long.
- Both the mouth and nose opens into the pharynx.
- It lies just posterior to the nasal cavity, oral cavity and larynx and just interior to the cervical vertebrae.
- Its wall is composed of skeletal muscles and lined with mucus membrane.
- Pharynx is divided into 3 parts:
  - ✓ **Nasopharynx:** The upper most part of the pharynx that lies posterior to the nasal cavity.
  - ✓ **Oropharynx:** The middle part of the pharynx that lies posterior to the oral cavity.
  - ✓ **Laryngopharynx**: The lowest portion of the pharynx that lies superior to the larynx.

Functions

- **Passageway for air and food**

  Pharynx is an organ involved in both the respiratory and digestive system. Air passes through nasal and oral section and food passes through oral and laryngeal sections.

- **Warming and humidifying the air**

  By the same methods as in the nose, the air is further warmed and moistened as it passes through the pharynx.

- **Taste**

  The olfactory nerve endings of the sense of taste are located in the epithelium of the oral and pharyngeal parts.

- **Protection**

  The lymphatic tissue of the pharyngeal and laryngeal tonsils produces antibodies in response to antigens.

- **Speech**

  The pharynx functions in speech by acting as a resonating chamber for sound. It helps to produce the voice.

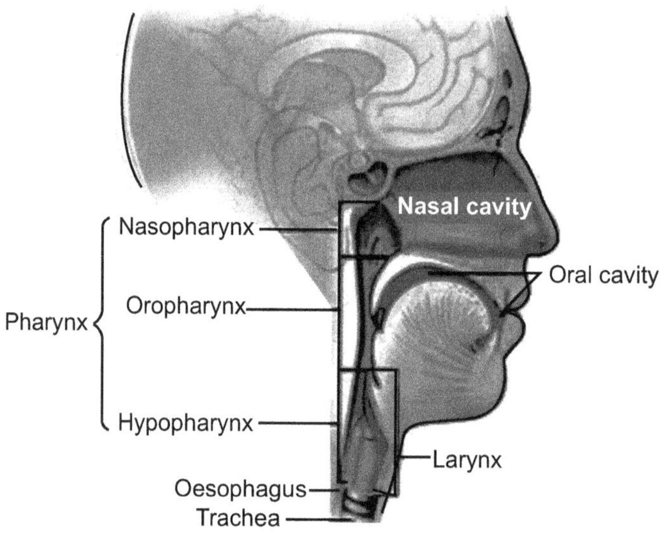

Fig. 4.3: Pharynx

Lower Respiratory System

4.6 LARYNX

- It is also called as voice box.
- It is a short passage that connects the pharynx with the trachea.
- The larynx is composed of irregular shaped cartilages attached to each other by ligaments and membranes.
- The main cartilages are:
  - ✓ Thyroid cartilages
  - ✓ Cricoid cartilage　　　　**Hyaline cartilage**
  - ✓ Arytenoid cartilage
  - ✓ Epiglottis: **Elastic cartilage**

Thyroid cartilage (Adam's apple)

- It consists of two fused plates of hyaline cartilage that forms anterior wall of the larynx which gives it a triangular shape.
- It is larger in males than in females.

Cricoid cartilage

- This lies below the thyroid cartilage.
- It is a ring of hyaline cartilage, attached to the 1st ring of trachea.
- It forms the inferior wall of the larynx.

Arytenoid cartilage

- These are the triangular pieces of hyaline cartilage
- It is located at the posterior of the cricoid cartilage.
- They provide attachment to the vocal cords.

Epiglottis

- It is a large leaf shaped piece of elastic cartilage.
- The stem of the epiglottis is attached to the thyroid cartilage but the leaf portion is unattached and free to move up and down like a trap door.
- If larynx is the voice box then epiglottis acts as a lid, it closes the larynx during swallowing and protects the lungs from entry of foreign objects.

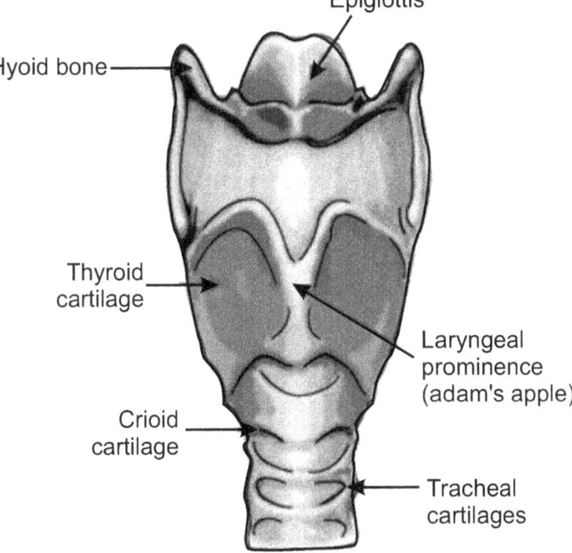

Fig. 4.4: Larynx

Functions of Larynx

- Production of sound
- Protection of the lower respiratory tract by ensuring that food passes into the oesophagus and not into the lower respiratory tract
- Acts as passageway for air
- It produces humidification, filtration and warming of air as it travels through the larynx.

4.7 PHYSIOLOGY OF VOICE PRODUCTION

- The vocal cords are two folds of mucus membrane with cord like free edges from thyroid cartilage anteriorly and arytenoid cartilage posteriorly.
- When the muscles controlling the vocal cords are relaxed, the vocal cords open and the passage way for air through the larynx is clear, the vocal cords are called as abducted (open vocal cords) (Figure 4.6)
- The pitch of sound produced by vibrating the vocal cords is low.
- When the muscle controlling the vocal cords contracts, the vocal cords are closed and the vocal cords are called as adducted (closed vocal cords) (Figure 4.7)
- The pitch of sound produced by such a vocal cord is high.
- When the vocal cords are stretched to this extent and are vibrated by air passing through it from the lungs, the sound produced is high pitched.
- The pitch of the voice is determined by the tension applied to the vocal cords through appropriate set of muscles.
- If they have pulled taut by the muscles, they vibrate more rapidly and a higher pitch results.
- The lower sound results by decreasing the tension on the vocal cords.

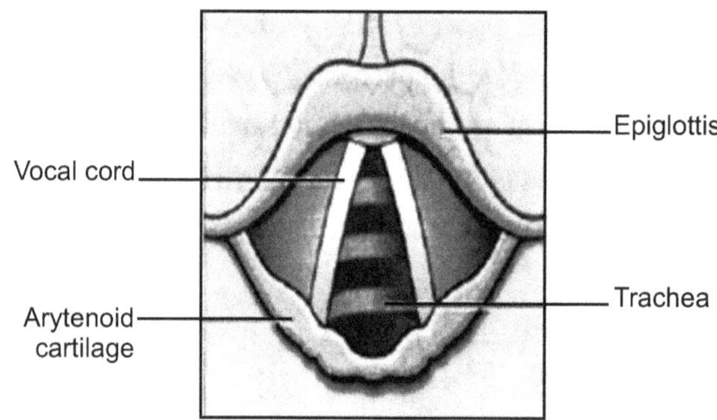

Fig. 4.5: Inferior view of the larynx

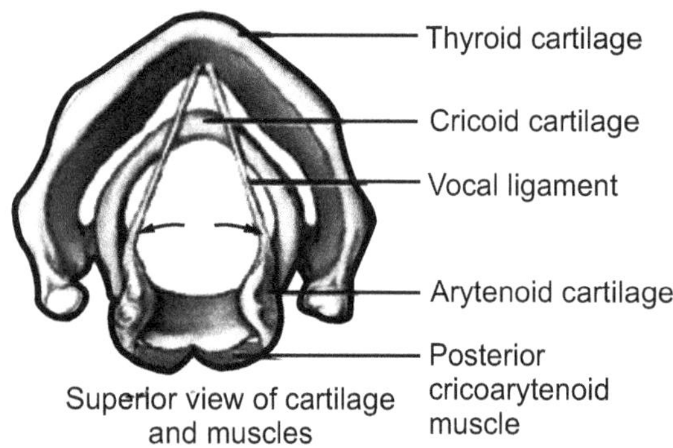

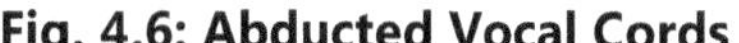

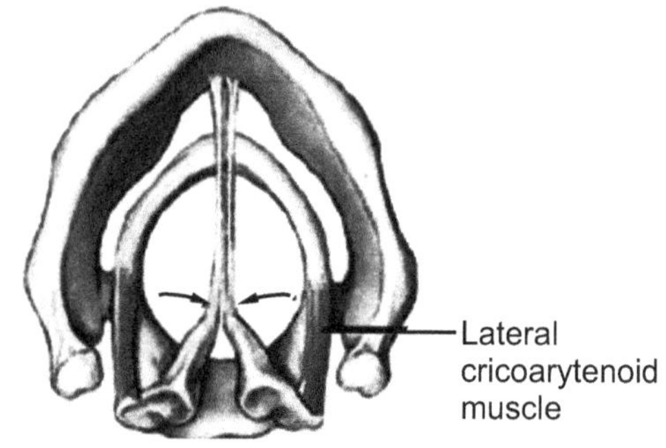

Fig. 4.6: Abducted Vocal Cords **Fig. 4.7: Adducted vocal cords**

4.8 TRACHEA (WIND PIPE)

- It is a tubular passageway for air.
- It is 12 cm long and 2.5 cm in diameter.
- It extends from the larynx to the 5th thoracic vertebrae where it divides into left and right primary bronchi.
- The trachea is located anterior to the oesophagus and has 'C' shaped cartilaginous rings within the wall.
- The trachea is made up of 4 main layers:
  - ✓ Adventitia (outer layer of areolar connective tissue)
  - ✓ The hyaline cartilage
  - ✓ The submucosa
  - ✓ The mucosa
- The mucosa is made up of pseudo-stratified ciliated columnar epithelium containing ciliated columnar cells, goblet cells and basal cells.
- The cilia move in a single direction thereby keeping the tract free of dust and particles.
- The single 'C' shaped cartilage ring provides a rigid support to the tracheal wall.
- At the point where the trachea divides into the right and left primary bronchi, there is an internal ridge called as carina.

Functions

- **Mucociliary escalator:** Mucus secreted by the goblet cells of mucosa moistens the air and traps the dust particles. The cilia moves the dust particles to the pharynx where they can be eliminated from the respiratory tract by expectoration (spitting).
- **Cough reflex:** A nerve ending in the larynx, trachea and bronchi are sensitive to the irritation which generates nerve impulses conducted by the vagus nerve to the respiratory centre in the brain stem.
- **Warming, humidifying and filtering of air:** Trachea produces humidification, filtration and warming of air as it travels through the trachea.

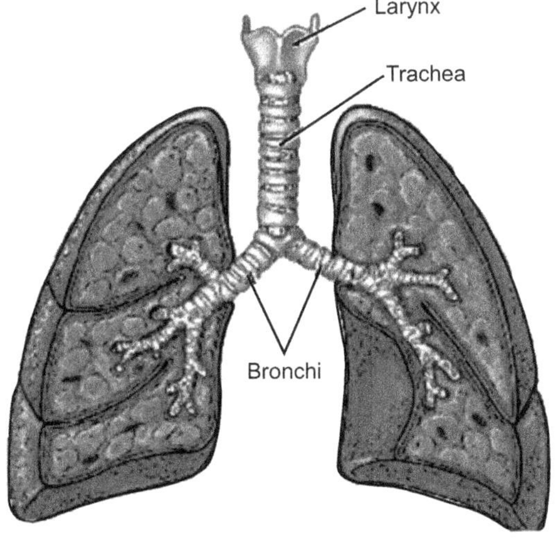

Fig. 4.8: Trachea and its associated structure

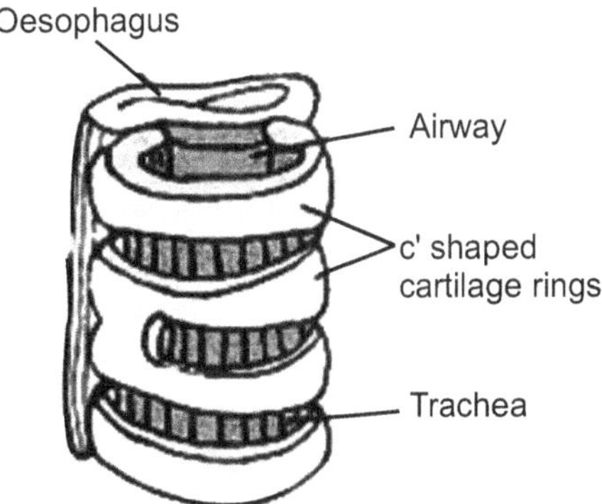

Fig. 4.9: 'C' shaped cartilaginous rings

4.9 LUNGS

- These are a pair of spongy, air-filled cone shaped organs located on either side of the chest (thorax).
- The lungs extend laterally from the heart to the ribs on both sides of the chest and continue posteriorly toward the spine.
- The superior end of the lung forms the cone and the inferior end forms the base.
- The left lung is slightly smaller than the right lung
- The right lung is thicker and broader than left lung
- The lungs are divided into;
    - ✓ **Apex:** The narrow superior portion of lung.
    - ✓ **Base:** The broad inferior portion of lung.
    - ✓ **Coastal surface:** The surface of lung lying against the ribs.
- **Medial surface:** It forms the lateral boundary of the mediastinum.
- The medial surface of each lung contains a region, the hilus through which the bronchi, pulmonary blood vessels, lymphatic vessels and nerves enter and exit.
- The lung is surrounded by two layers of delicate serous membrane called as pleural membrane.
- The inner membrane which covers the lungs is called as visceral pleura and the outer layer which is attached to the wall of thoracic cavity is called as parietal pleura.
- The space between these two layers called as pleural cavity contains, lubricating fluid secreted by membranes.
- This fluid reduces friction between the membranes and allows them to move easily on one another during breathing.

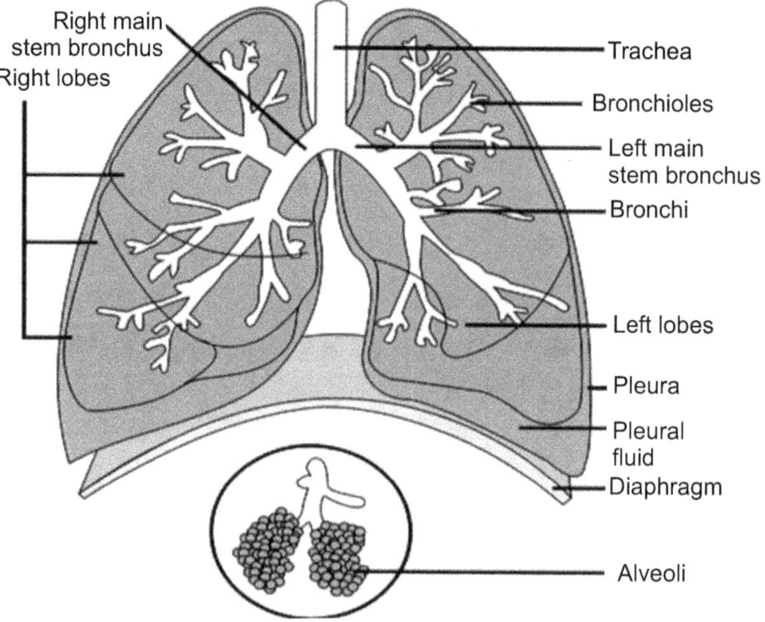

Fig. 4.10: Lung

Lobes of lungs
- The right lung is subdivided into 3 lobes:
  - ✓ Superior lobe
  - ✓ Middle lobe
  - ✓ Inferior lobe
- The left lung is subdivided into 2 lobes:
  - ✓ Superior lobe
  - ✓ Inferior lobe

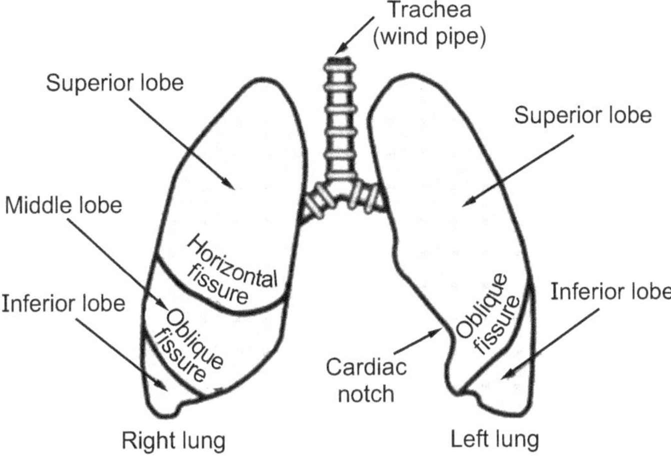

Fig. 4.11: Lobes of lungs

Fissures of lungs
- Fissures are double-fold of visceral pleura that either completely or incompletely invaginate lung parenchyma to form the lung lobes.
- **Right lung:** It has two fissures:
  - ✓ **Oblique fissure:** It separates the upper lobes from the lower lobes
  - ✓ **Horizontal fissure:** It separates the right upper lobe from the right middle lobe
- **Left lung:** It has one fissure:
  - ✓ **Oblique fissure:** It separates superior lobe and inferior lobe.

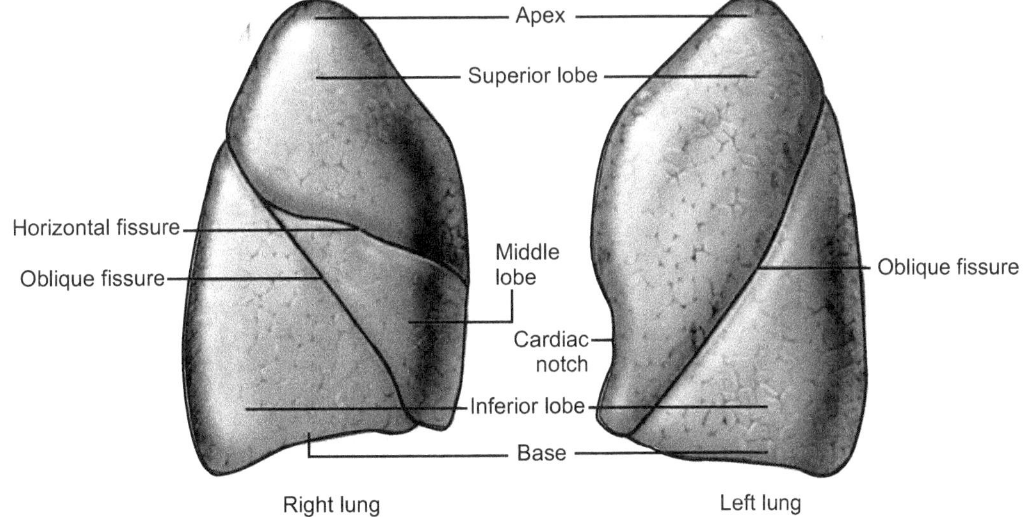

Fig. 4.12: Fissures of lung

4.10 BRONCHI

- At the level of fifth thoracic vertebra, the trachea divides into right pulmonary bronchus which goes into right lung and left pulmonary bronchus which goes into left lung.
- Bronchi are large, hollow tubes made of hyaline cartilage lined with ciliated pseudostratified epithelium.

Right bronchus

- It is wider, shorter and more vertical than left bronchus.
- It is 2.5 cm long.
- After entering the right lung at hilum it is (primary bronchi) divided into 3 secondary bronchi, one for each lobe of lung.

Left bronchus

- It is 5 cm long and narrower than the right bronchus.
- After entering the left lung it divides into 2 secondary bronchi, one for each lobe of lung.
- The secondary bronchi further divides into smaller bronchi called as tertiary bronchi that divide into bronchioles.
- Bronchioles further divides into smaller bronchioles to form tube called as terminal bronchioles.
- Terminal bronchioles further divide into the respiratory bronchioles.

Functions

- The primary function is the control of air entering the lungs.
- The diameter of respiratory system is altered by contraction or relaxation, thus regulating the volume of air entering the lungs.

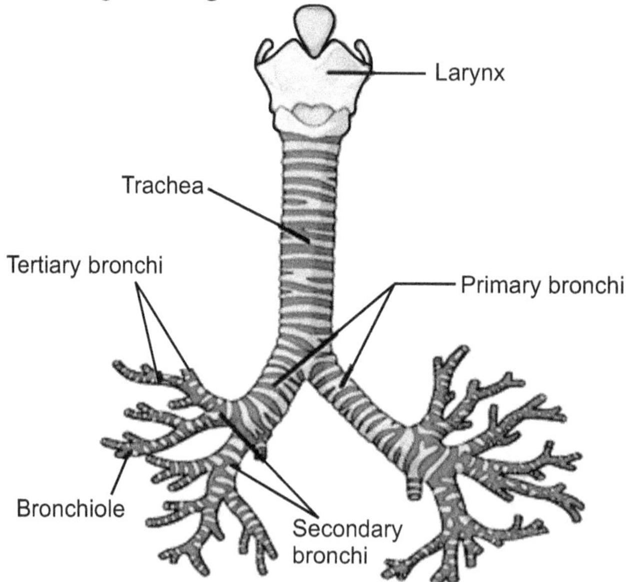

Fig. 4.13: Bronchi

4.11 LOBULES

- Each lobe of lung is divided into many small compartments called as lobules.
- Each lobule is covered by elastic connective tissue and contains lymphatic vessels, an arteriole, a venule and a branch from a terminal bronchiole.
- Terminal bronchioles are subdivided into microscopic branches called as respiratory bronchioles.
- Respiratory bronchioles in turn are subdivided into several (2-11) alveolar ducts.
- The alveolar ducts are surrounded by alveoli and alveoli sacs.
- The alveoli are cup- shaped structures and surrounded by the capillary network.
- The alveolar wall consists of two types of cells.
- **Type 1 alveolar cells:** It forms a lining of alveolar wall.
- **Type 2 alveolar cells:** It secretes alveolar fluid (complex mixture of phospholipids and lipoproteins), which keeps the alveolar cells moist.

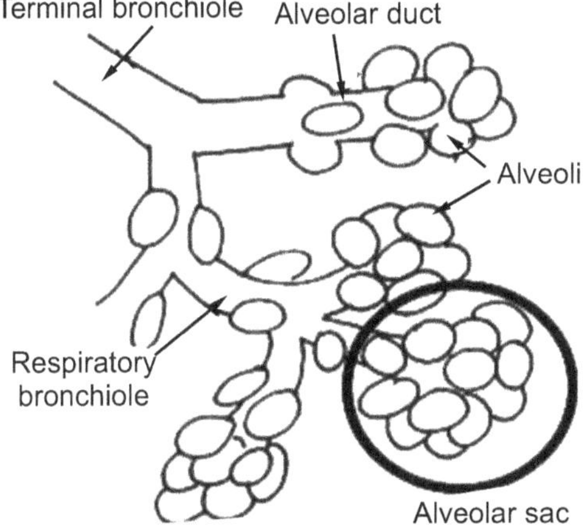

Fig. 4.14: Alveolar duct and sac

4.12 PHYSIOLOGY OF RESPIRATION

Respiration is divided into two phases, external and internal respiration.

External Respiration (Pulmonary gas exchange)

- It is the exchange of gases between the air spaces of the lungs and the blood in pulmonary capillaries.
- In this process, pulmonary capillary blood gains O_2 and loses CO_2.
- Right ventricle: It pumps deoxygenated blood to the lungs for purification.
- Left ventricle: It pumps oxygenated blood to all other parts of the body.
- External respiration or pulmonary gas exchange is the diffusion of O_2 from air in the alveoli of the lungs to blood in the pulmonary capillaries and the diffusion of CO_2 in the opposite direction.
- External respiration in the lungs convert deoxygenated blood coming from the right side of the heart into oxygenated blood that returns to the left side of the heart.
- As blood flows through the pulmonary capillaries it picks up O_2 from alveolar air and unloads CO_2 into alveolar air.

- This process is called as exchange of gases; each gas diffuses independently from the area where partial pressure is low.
- O_2 diffuses from alveolar air, where its partial pressure is 105 mm Hg into the blood in pulmonary capillaries, where P_{CO2} is only 40 mm Hg in resting person.
- In a person who is exercising the P_{O2} will be even lower because contracting muscle fibres are using more O_2.
- Diffusion continues until the P_{O2} of pulmonary capillary blood increases to match the P_{O2} of alveolar air, 105 mm Hg.
- While O_2 is diffusing from alveolar air into the deoxygenated blood, CO_2 is diffusing in opposite direction.
- The P_{CO2} of deoxygenated blood is 45 mm Hg in a resting person, whereas P_{CO2} of alveolar air is 40 mm Hg.
- Because of this difference in P_{CO2}, carbon dioxide diffuses from deoxygenated blood into the alveoli until the P_{CO2} of the blood decreases to 40 mm Hg.
- Thus the P_{O2} and P_{CO2} of oxygenated blood leaving the lungs are same as in the alveolar air.
- The CO_2 that diffuses into the alveoli is eliminated from the lungs during expiration.

Rate of external respiration depends on several factors which are given below.

Partial pressure difference

- As the alveolar P_{O2} is higher that P_{O2} in a systemic vein, O_2 diffuses from the alveoli into the blood.
- As a person goes at high altitude, the atmospheric P_{O2} decreases, the alveolar P_{O2} also decreases and less O_2 diffuses into the blood.

Surface area for gas exchange

- The surface area for diffusion of gas is large (about 70 m^2).
- Any pulmonary disorder that decreases the functional surface area decreases the rate of external respiration.

Diffusion distance

- The total thickness of alveolar capillary membrane is 0.5 µm.
- Thicker the membrane slower is the rate of diffusion.

Breathing rate and depth

- External respiration also depends on average rate of airflow into and out of the lungs.

Internal Respiration (Systemic Gas Exchange)

- It is the exchange of gases between the blood in systemic capillary and the systemic tissue cells.
- In this process the systemic capillary gains CO_2 and loses O_2.
- Internal respiration results in the conversion of oxygenated blood to deoxygenated blood.
- Oxygenated blood entering the tissue capillaries has a P_{O2} of 100 mm Hg, whereas tissue cells have an average of P_{O2} of 40 mm Hg.
- Because of this difference in P_{O2}, oxygen diffuses from the oxygenated blood through interstitial fluid and into tissue cells until the P_{O2} in the blood decreases to 40 mm Hg.

- This is average P_{O_2} of deoxygenated blood entering tissue when one is at rest.
- While O_2 diffuses from the blood capillaries into the tissue cells, CO_2 diffuses in the opposite direction.
- The average P_{CO_2} of tissue cells is 45 mm Hg whereas, tissue capillary oxygenated blood is 40 mm Hg.
- As a result CO_2 diffuses from tissue cells through interstitial fluid into the oxygenated blood until the Pco_2 in the blood increases to 45 mm Hg, the P_{CO_2} of tissue capillary deoxygenated blood.
- From here the deoxygenated blood returns to the heart and it is pumped to the lungs for another cycle of external respiration.

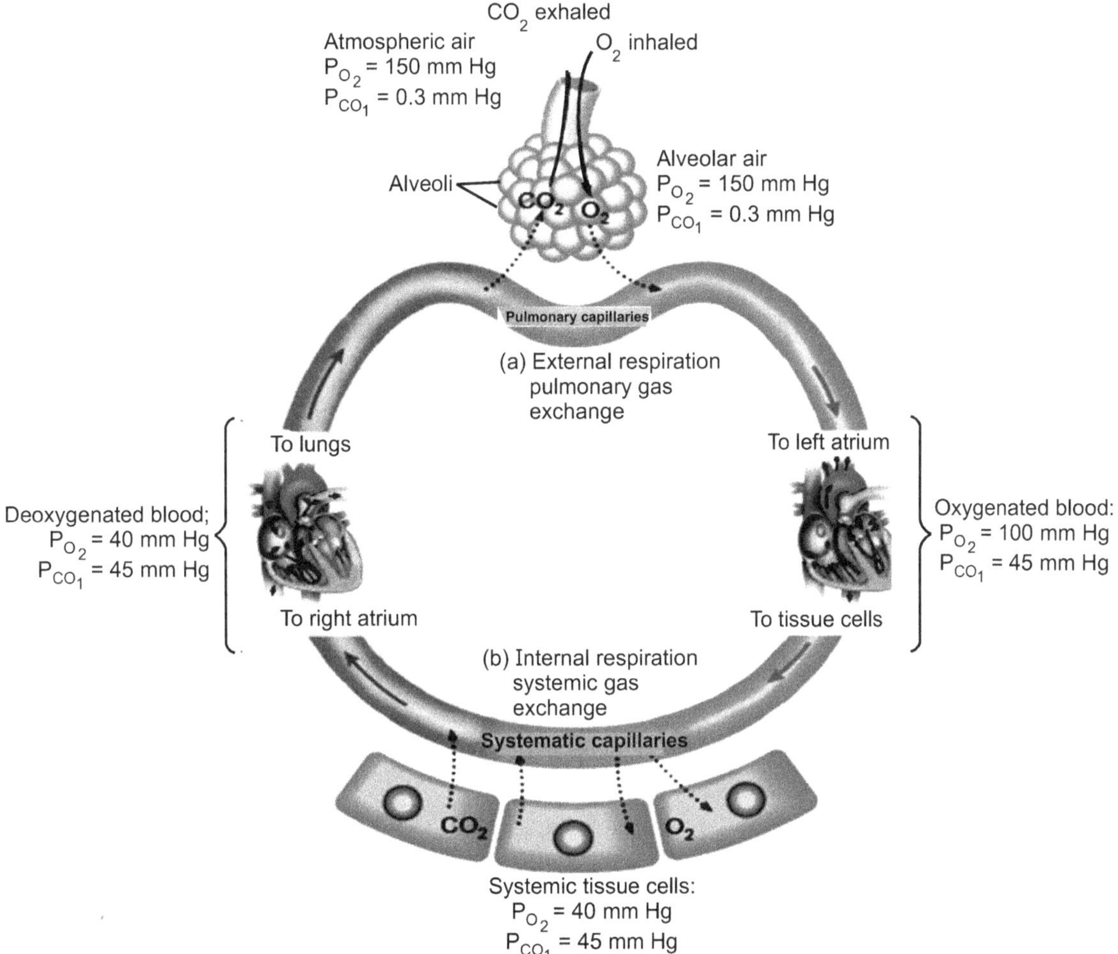

Fig. 4.15: Physiology of Respiration

4.13 TRANSPORT OF OXYGEN AND CARBON DIOXIDE

- When O_2 and CO_2 enter the blood, certain chemical reactions occur that results in gas transport and gas exchange.
- Transport of gases between the lungs and the body tissues is a function of blood.

OXYGEN

- O_2 does not dissolve easily in water; only about 1.5 % is dissolved in the blood plasma.
- About 98.5% of O_2 transported to Hb, combines with it inside the red blood cells.
- Each 100 ml of oxygenated blood contains about 20 ml of oxygen, 0.3 ml dissolved in plasma and 19.7 ml bound to haemoglobin.
- Haemoglobin (Hb) consists of two parts, a protein called as globin and an iron containing protein called as heme.
- O_2 and Hb combines in reversible reaction to form oxyhaemoglobin as follows:

$$\text{Hb} \quad + \quad O_2 \quad \underset{\text{Dissociation of } O_2}{\overset{\text{Binding of } O_2}{\rightleftharpoons}} \quad \text{Hb} - O_2$$

Reduced hemoglobin   Oxygen

(deoxyhemoglobin)   Oxyhemoglobin

- 98.5% of the O_2 is bound to haemoglobin and is the trapped inside the RBCs, only dissolved O_2 (1.5%) can diffuse out of tissue capillaries into cells.

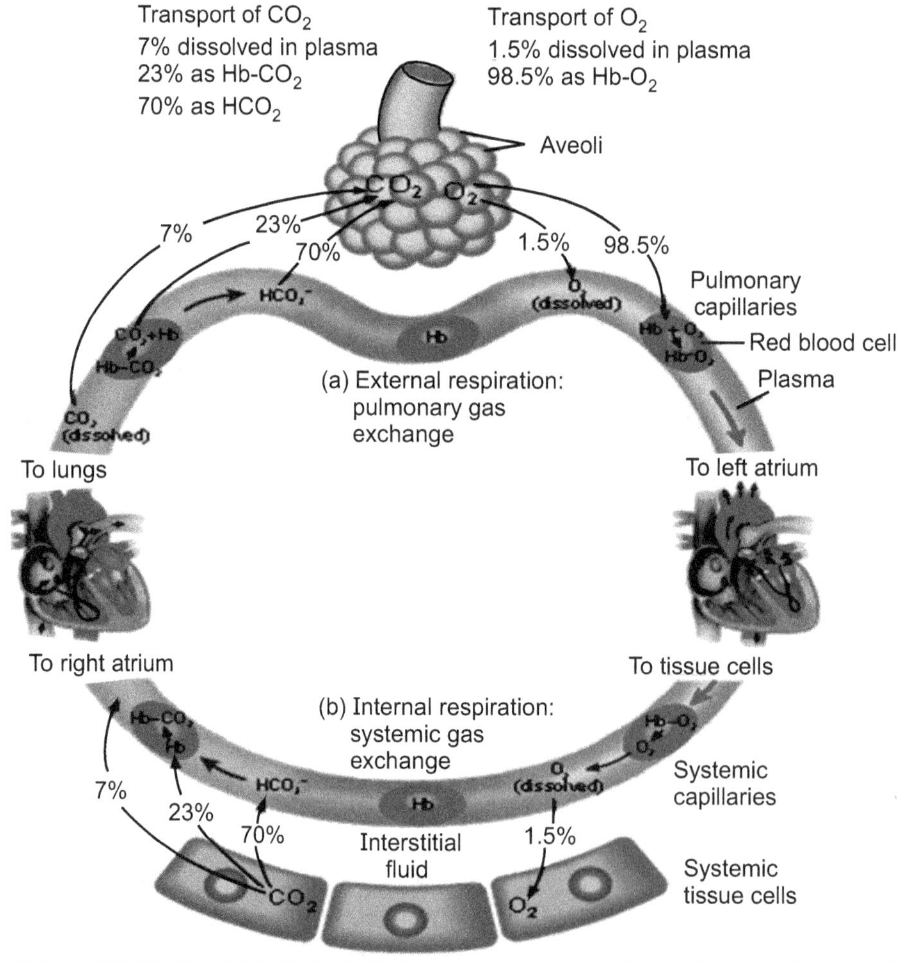

Fig. 4.16: Transport of gases

Factors affecting Hb and O_2 Binding

- Greater the P_{O2}, the more oxygen will combine with Hb.
- Lesser the P_{O2}, lesser oxygen will combine with Hb.

Hb and acidity (pH):

- As acidity increases (pH decreases), the affinity of haemoglobin for O_2 decreases and O_2 dissociates more readily from the haemoglobin.
- In acidic environment, Hb affinity for O_2 is lower and oxygen splits more rapidly from Hb. This is called as Bohr Effect.
- The Bohr effect works in both ways: An increase in H^+ ions in blood causes O_2 to unload from haemoglobin and the binding of O_2 to haemoglobin causes unloading of H^+ ions from haemoglobin.

Partial pressure of CO_2

- As P_{CO2} rises, Hb releases O_2 more readily.
- Low blood pH (acidic condition) results from high CO_2.
- As CO_2 is taken up by the blood, it is converted to carbonic acid with the help of enzyme carbonic acid anhydrase in red blood cells.

$$CO_2 \; + \; H_2O \; \overset{CA}{\rightleftharpoons} \; H_2CO_3 \; \rightleftharpoons \; H^+ \; + \; HCO_3^-$$

| Carbon dioxide | Water | | Carbonic acid | | Hydrogen ion | | Bicarbonate ion |

- Thus, carbonic acid formed in RBC's dissociates in H^+ and HCO_3^-.
- As the H^+ ions concentration increases pH decreases.
- Thus, increased P_{CO2} produce a more acidic environment that helps to split O_2 from Hb.

Temperature

- As temperature increases, the oxygen is released from the haemoglobin.

2, 3-biphosphoglycerate (BPG)

- A substance found in RBC called as BPG decreases the affinity of Hb for O_2 and thus help to release O_2 from haemoglobin.

Foetal haemoglobin

- Foetal Hb differs from adult Hb in structure and in its affinity for oxygen.
- Foetal Hb has a higher affinity for O_2 because it binds to BPG less strongly.

CARBON DIOXIDE

- Each 100 ml of deoxygenated blood contains 5 ml of CO_2 which is carried by blood in 3 main forms.
- **Dissolved CO_2:** 7% is dissolved in plasma. Upon reaching the lungs, it diffuses into the lungs.
- **Carbaminohaemoglobin:** 23% combines with the globin portion of Hb to form carbaminoglobin. The formation of Hb-CO_2 is greatly influenced by P_{CO2}.

$$Hb \; + \; CO_2 \; \rightleftharpoons \; Hb - CO_2$$

Hemoglobin Carbon dioxide Carbaminohemoglobin

Bicarbonate ions:

- 70% is transported in plasma as bicarbonate ions.
- As CO_2 diffuses into tissue capillaries and enters RBC it reacts with water in the presence of an enzyme carbonic anhydrase to form carbonic acid.
- The carbonic acid dissociates to form H^+ and HCO_3^-.
- Many of H^+ ions combine with Hb to form H. Hb and bicarbonate ions accumulates inside the RBCs.

$$CO_2 \;+\; H_2O \; \overset{\text{Carbonic anhydrase}}{\rightleftharpoons} \; H_2CO_3 \; \rightleftharpoons \; H^+ \;+\; HCO_3^-$$

Carbon dioxide   Water   Carbonic acid   Hydrogen ion   Bicarbonate ion

4.14 PULMONARY VOLUMES AND CAPACITIES

During the process of normal breathing about 500 ml of air moves into the respiratory passageway with each inspiration and moves out with each expiration.

- ✓ **Tidal volume (TV):** This is the amount of air passing in and out of lungs during each cycle of breathing (15 cycles/min).
- ✓ **Inspiratory reserve volume (IRV) (3100 ml):** This is the extra volume of air that can be inhaled into the lungs during maximal inspiration. i.e. above normal TV.
- ✓ **Expiratory reserve volume (ERV) (1200 ml):** This is the largest volume of air which can be expelled from the lungs during maximal expiration.
- ✓ **Residual volume (RV) (1200 ml):** It is the volume of air remaining in the lungs after forced expiration.
- ✓ **Inspiratory capacity (IC) (3600 ml):** It is the sum of Tidal volume + Inspiratory reserve volume.
- ✓ **Functional residual (FRC) (2400 ml):** It is the sum of Residual volume + Expiratory reserve volume.
- ✓ **Vital capacity (VC) (4800 ml):** This is the maximum volume of air which can be moved on and out of the lungs (Tidal volume + IRV+ ERV)
- ✓ **Total lung capacity (6000 ml):** It is the sum of all volume (TV + IRV + ERV + RV).
- Spirogram is the most common pulmonary function test which specifically measures the amount (volume) and the speed (flow) of air that can be inhaled and exhaled from the lungs.
- A spirometer is a volume recorder consisting of a double-walled cylinder with an inverted bell immersed in water to form a seal.
- When air enters the spirometer from the lungs, the bell rises.
- A downward deflection represents expiration and an upward deflection represents inspiration.
- The slope of the spirogram measures the rate of airflow and the amplitude of the deflection measures the volume of air.
- Volume is plotted on the vertical axis (y axis) and time is plotted on the horizontal axis (x axis).

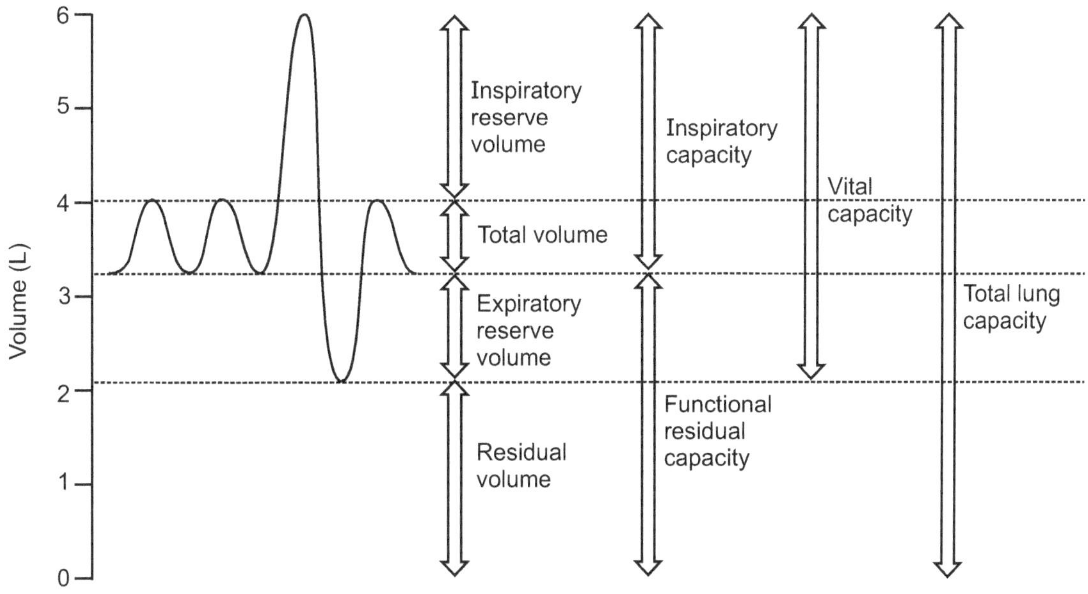

Fig. 4.17: Spirogram

4.15 ARTIFICIAL RESPIRATIONS AND RESUSCITATION METHODS

- Artificial ventilation also called as artificial respiration.
- It is any means of assisting or stimulating respiration, a metabolic process referring to the overall exchange of gases in the body by pulmonary ventilation, external respiration and internal respiration.
- The air may be provided manually to a person who is not breathing or is not making sufficient respiratory effort on his/her own or it may be mechanical ventilation involving the use of a mechanical ventilator to move air in and out of the lungs.

Types of artificial respiration:

- There are four types:
  - ✓ Manual methods
  - ✓ Mechanical methods
  - ✓ Cardiopulmonary resuscitation
  - ✓ Oxygen therapy

Manual methods:

- It is achieved through manual insufflation of the lungs either by the rescuer blowing into the patient's lungs (mouth-to-mouth resuscitation).
- Two types of respiration:
  - ✓ Mouth to mouth respiration
  - ✓ Mouth to nose respiration

Mouth to mouth respiration:

- It is also called as artificial respiration.
- Pinch the nose of patient with one hand so as to open mouth and breathe in a lungful of air.

- Then tightly seal the mouth with the patients open mouth and breathe out forcefully into his mouth.
- Now move up, inhale more air from the atmosphere, again seal the mouth with patient's mouth, pinch his nose and breathe out into him forcefully.
- Go on repeating the same procedure rapidly for number of times so as to saturate the patient's blood with oxygen.
- At the same time watch if the lungs of the patients are expanding and falling.
- The air we breathe in contains 20% oxygen while the expired air contains 16% oxygen.
- Give 12 breathings per minute to an adult patient.

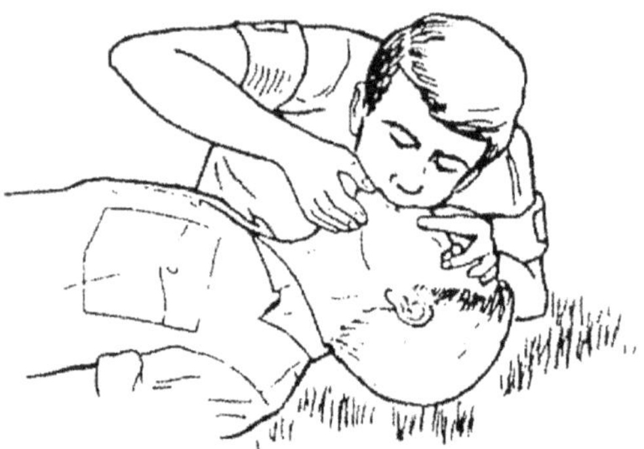

Fig. 4.18: Mouth to mouth respiration

Mouth to nose respiration:
- If we are unable to open the mouth of the patient due to fracture of jaw or due to some other reason than we should start mouth to nose respiration.
- For mouth to nose respiration seal the mouth with patient's nose and do the same procedure as in case of mouth to mouth respiration.

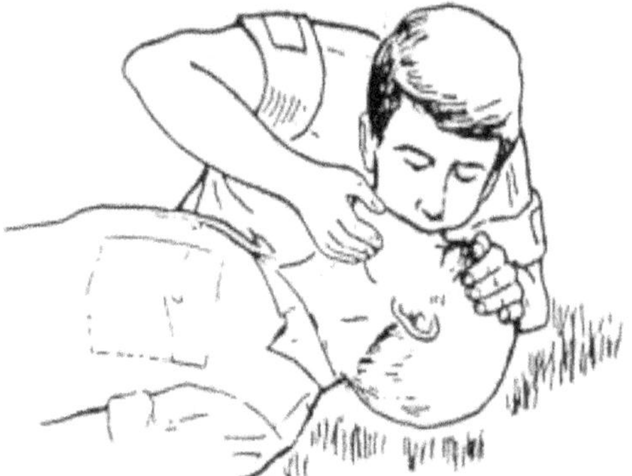

Fig. 4.19: Mouth to nose respiration

Mechanical methods:
- This method mechanically assists or replaces spontaneous breathing.
- It may involve a machine called as ventilator by a registered nurse, physician, physician assistant, respiratory therapist, paramedic or other suitable person.
- There are two modes of mechanical ventilation:
- ***Positive pressure ventilation***: In this air is pushed into the trachea
- ***Negative pressure ventilation:*** In this air is sucked into the lungs.

Cardio-pulmonary resuscitation (CPR):

- It is an emergency procedure, performed in an effort to manually preserve intact brain function until further measures are taken to restore spontaneous blood circulation and breathing in a person in cardiac arrest.
- It is indicated in unresponsive patients with no breathing or abnormal breathing.
- CPR alone is unlikely to restart the heart.
- Its main purpose is to restore partial flow of oxygenated blood to the brain and heart.
- The objective is to delay the tissue death and to extend the brief window of opportunity for a successful resuscitation without permanent brain damage.
- CPR may succeed in inducing a heart rhythm which may be shockable.
- CPR is generally continued until the patient has a return of spontaneous circulation or is declared dead.
- CPR consists of artificial respiration and artificial circulation.
- As soon as heart stops beating and breathing also stops, the person is considered clinically dead but the vital centers like brain remain viable for 4-6 minutes.
- If during this period CPR is given the life of patient may be revived.
- CPR can be performed under following steps.
- It can be done by ABC formula.
  A = Airway clearance
  B = Breathing
  C = Circulation or cardiac massage

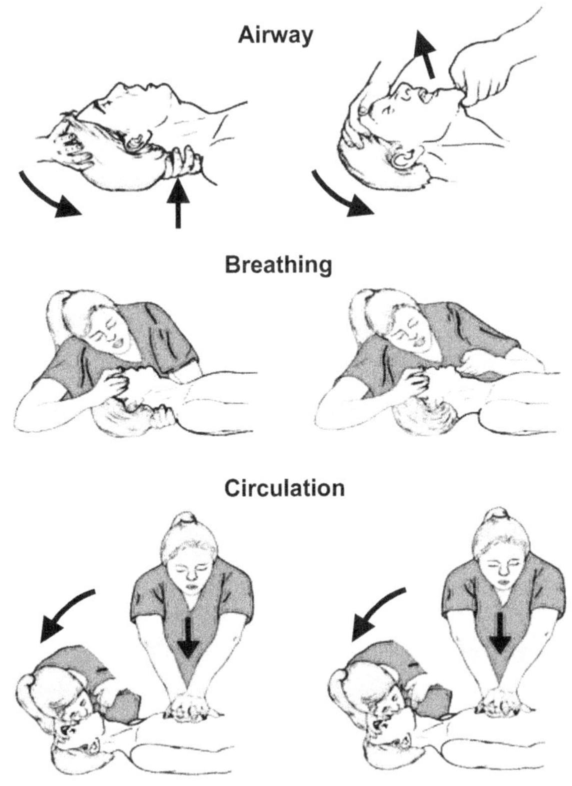

Fig. 4.20: CPR process

A = Airway (Clear the airway):

- First of all the air passages should be opened and cleaned so as to make a free passage for air.
- For this purpose wrap a handkerchief or a piece of clean cloth on first two fingers together and clean victim's mouth taking care that his breathing is not blocked.
- During cleaning process the mouth of the patient should be turned to a side so that the particles of cleaned material may not fall in the respiratory tract.

B = Breathing

- Without food a person can survive for 70 days, without water for 7 days but without oxygen a person cannot survive for more than 3-4 minutes.
- If the breathing has stopped, then after clearing of the airways immediately start giving respiration.

C = Circulation or cardiac massage:

- If the heart stops beating which can be diagnosed by loss of consciousness, absence of pulse rate feeling at the wrist then cardiac massage should be started at once to revive the heart beat so as to circulate the blood to various organs of the body including brain.
- Place the victim horizontally on the ground or on a flat, hard surface with face in the upward position.
- Kneel on the side of the chest of the victim.
- Place the right hand two fingers above the lower end of the sternum.
- Place the left hand over the right hand.
- At this place press the breast bone down towards the spine for about 4 minutes, 4 cm in an adult.
- After applying pressure for about half second releases the pressure after each compression, completely relax the pressure so that the sternum returns to the normal position. Compression and relaxation time should be equal.
- Repeat the cycle 60-70 times a minute for an adult.
- If the breathing and heart beating both are absent then immediately start artificial breathing and external cardiac massage together in a rhythmic manner.
- After every 5 heart compression, one mouth to mouth breathing should be given to the patient.
- The cycle is repeated until the breathing and heart beating comes to normal.
- If the treatment is effective the following signs will appear.
- Colour of face and skin will become normal.
- Pupil will start contracting.
- Pulsation and heart beating will be felt.

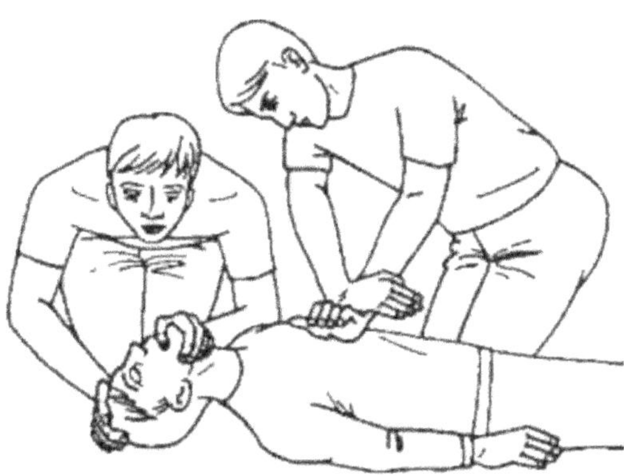

Fig. 4.21: Cardiac massage

Oxygen therapy:

- It is also known as supplemental oxygen, is the use of oxygen as a medical treatment.
- This can be used for low blood oxygen, carbon monoxide toxicity and to maintain enough oxygen while inhaled anesthetics are given.

4.16 DISORDERS OF THE RESPIRATORY SYSTEM

Pneumonia

- It is an acute infection or inflammation of the alveoli.
- When certain microbes enter the lungs of susceptible individuals, they release damaging toxins, stimulating inflammation and immune responses that have damaging side-effects.
- The toxins and immune response damage alveoli and bronchial mucous membrane, inflammation and edema of alveoli, interfering with ventilation and gas exchange.
- Most common cause of pneumonia is the pneumococcal bacterium i.e. *Streptococcus pneumoniae.*

Tuberculosis

- The bacterium *Mycobacterium tuberculosis* is the causative agent of an infectious communicable disease called as tuberculosis that most often affect the lungs and the pleura but may involve other parts of the body.
- Once the bacteria enter the lungs, they multiply and cause inflammation, which stimulates the neutrophils and macrophages to migrate to the area and engulf the bacteria to prevent their spread.
- Symptoms are fatigue, weight loss, lethargy, anorexia, a low grade fever, night sweats, cough, dyspnoea, chest pain and hemolysis.

Coryza and Influenza

- Many viruses can cause coryza (common cold) but a group of viruses called as rhinoviruses are responsible for about 40% of all colds.
- Symptoms are sneezing, excessive nasal secretion, dry cough and congestion.

- Complications include sinusitis, asthma, bronchitis, ear infections and laryngitis.
- Influenza (flu) is also caused by virus.
- Symptoms includes chills, fever (usually higher than 39°C), headache and muscular aches.

Pulmonary edema

- It is an abnormal accumulation of fluid in the interstitial spaces and alveoli of lungs.
- Edema may arise from increased permeability of pulmonary capillaries.
- Most common symptoms are dyspnoea.
- Others symptoms are wheezing, rapid breathing rate, restlessness, a feeling of suffocation, cyanosis, paleness, excessive perspiration and pulmonary hypertension.

Cystic fibrosis

- It is an inherited disease of secretory epithelia that affects the airways, liver, pancreas, small intestine and sweat glands.
- It is characterised by abnormal transport of chloride and sodium across an epithelium, leading to thick and viscous secretions.

Asthma

- It is a disorder characterised by chronic airway inflammation, airway hyper sensitivity to a variety of stimuli and airway obstruction.
- The trigger for asthma is an allergen such as pollen, house dust mites, molds, or particular food.
- Other common triggers of asthma are emotional distress, aspirin, sulfiting agents (used in wine and beer), exercise and breathing cold air or cigarette smoke.
- The symptoms include difficulty in breathing, coughing, wheezing, chest congestion, tachycardia, fatigue and anxiety.

Chronic Obstructive Pulmonary Disease (COPD)

- It is a type of respiratory disease characterised by chronic and recurrent obstruction of airflow which increases the airway resistance.
- COPD are of 2 types:
  - Emphysema
  - Chronic bronchitis
  - ✓ **Emphysema:** It is a disorder characterised by destruction of the alveoli walls producing abnormally large air spaces that remain filled with air during exhalation. It is caused by long term irritation, cigarette smoke, air pollution and occupational exposure to industrial dust.
  - ✓ **Chronic bronchitis:** It is a disorder characterised by excessive secretion of bronchial mucus. Cigarette smoking is the main cause. Symptoms are productive cough (sputum), shortness of breath, wheezing, cyanosis, pulmonary hypertension.

Lung cancer

- In the United States lung cancer is the leading cause of cancer deaths; both in males and females.
- Cigarette smoking is identified as one of the major cause of lung cancer.
- The most common type of lung cancer is bronchiogenic carcinoma which starts in the epithelium of the bronchial tubes.
- Symptoms are chronic cough, spitting blood from respiratory tract, wheezing, shortness of breath, chest pain, hoarseness, difficulty in swallowing, weight loss, anorexia, fatigue, bone pain, headache, anaemia, jaundice and thrombocytopenia.

Asbestos related disease

- These are serious lung cancer disorders that develop due to inhalation of asbestos particles.
- When they are inhaled they penetrate the lung tissue.
- However, the fibres usually destroy the white blood cells and scarring of lung tissue may follow.
- Asbestos-related diseases include asbestosis (widespread scarring of lung tissue), diffuse pleural thickening (thickening of the pleurae), and mesothelioma (cancer of the pleurae or the peritoneum).

QUESTIONS

Short Answer Questions

1. Define respiration.
2. Enlist different processes of respiration.
3. Classify respiratory system.
4. Write a note on structure and function of lungs.
5. Draw well labeled diagram of respiratory system.
6. Define the terms: (i) Acute bronchitis (ii) Chronic bronchitis (iii) Asthma
7. Explain the physiology of voice production.
8. Explain transport of O_2 and CO_2.
9. Explain the various techniques of artificial respiration.

Long Answer Questions

1. Draw well labeled diagram of spirogram and explain various pulmonary volumes and capacities.
2. Describe gross anatomy of lungs. Explain exchange of gases at alveolar and cellular level.

3. Enlist different organs involved in respiration. Explain mechanism of breathing and exchange of gases at lung and tissue level.

4. Draw a neat labeled diagram of human respiratory system. Explain in detail transport of O_2 and CO_2 during respiration.

5. Define respiration. Explain in detail mechanism of breathing and exchange of gases during respiration.

Chapter 5

URINARY SYSTEM

♦ LEARNING OBJECTIVES ♦

❖ To describe the internal structure of kidney.

❖ To list different functions of the kidneys.

❖ To study the structure and function of nephron.

❖ To describe the physiology of urine formation.

❖ To define urinalysis and give its importance.

❖ To define renal plasma clearance and give its importance.

❖ To describe the anatomy and physiology of the ureters, urinary bladder, and urethra.

❖ To describe the micturition reflex.

❖ To describe the water balance and electrolyte balance.

5.1 INTRODUCTION

Nephrology is a branch of medicine that concerns with the study of kidney function, kidney disease, their treatment and renal replacement therapy (dialysis and kidney transplantation).

The branch of medicine that deals with male and female urinary systems called as urology. Urinary system is also called as renal system.

- The purpose of the renal system is to eliminate waste from the body, regulate blood volume and pressure, control the levels of electrolytes and metabolites and regulate blood pH.

- The urinary system consists of two kidneys, ureters, urinary bladder and urethra

- The kidneys secrete urine.

- The ureters convey the urine from the kidneys to the urinary bladder.

- The urinary bladder collects and stores urine temporarily.

- The urethra discharges the urine formed by the kidney to the exterior of body.

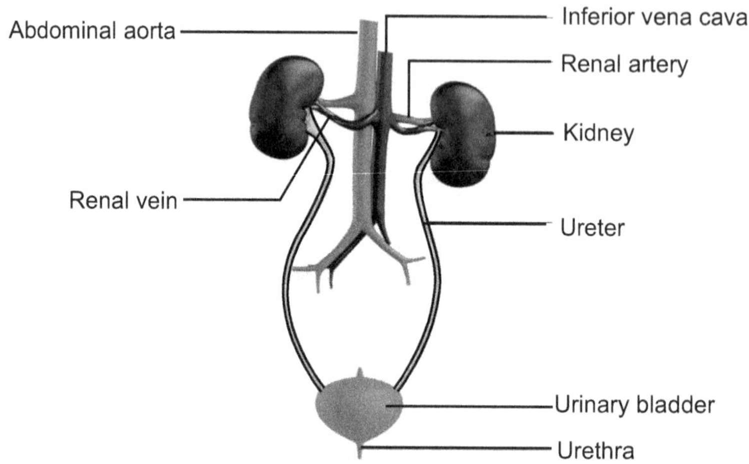

Fig. 5.1: Urinary System

5.2 KIDNEYS

External Anatomy of Kidney

- These are paired, reddish, bean shaped organs.
- The right kidney is slightly lower than the left kidney.
- The typical kidney is 10-12 cm long, 5-7 cm wide and 3 cm thick.
- It has a mass of 135-150 gm.
- Near the centre of concave border of kidney is a deep, vertical fissure called as renal hilus.
- Through the hilus of the kidneys, the ureters emerge along with the blood vessels, lymphatic vessels and nerves.
- Externally the kidneys are surrounded by three layers.
  - ✓ **Renal fascia:** Outer layer, made up of dense irregular connective tissue.
  - ✓ **Adipose capsule:** Middle layer is a mass of fatty tissue. It protects the kidneys from trauma and holds it firmly in place in the abdominal cavity.
  - ✓ **Renal capsule:** Inner layer, made up of dense irregular connective tissue. It is continuous with the outer layer of the ureter. It serves as a barrier against trauma and helps maintain the shape of the kidney.

Internal Anatomy of Kidney

The kidney is divided into two sections:
  - ✓ **Renal cortex:** It is the superficial, smooth textured reddish area.
  - ✓ **Renal medulla:** It is the deep, reddish brown inner region.
- The renal medulla consists of 8 to 18 cone shaped renal pyramids.
- The base (wider end) of each pyramid faces the renal cortex and apex (narrower end) called as renal papilla points towards the renal hilus.

- The renal cortex is a smooth area extending from the renal capsule to the bases of renal pyramids and into the spaces between them.
- Those portions of the renal cortex that extend between the renal pyramids are called as renal columns.
- A renal lobe consists of a renal pyramid, its overlying area of renal cortex and one half of each adjacent renal column.
- Together, the renal cortex and renal pyramids of the renal medulla constitute the parenchyma of the kidney.
- The parenchyma contains the functional units of the kidney called as nephrons.
- Urine formed by the nephrons drains into large papillary ducts which extend through the renal papillae of the pyramids.
- The papillary ducts drain into cuplike structures called as minor and major calyces.
- Each kidney has 8 to 18 minor calyces and 2 to 3 major calyces.
- A minor calyx receives urine from the papillary ducts of one renal papilla and delivers to a major calyx.
- From the major calyx, urine drains into a single large cavity called as renal pelvis and then out through the ureter to the urinary bladder.
- The hilus expands into a cavity within the kidney called as renal sinus which contains part of the renal pelvis, the calyces and branches of the renal blood vessels and nerves.

Functions
- It regulates water balance and various inorganic ions.
- It removes the metabolic waste products from the blood and excretes them into the urine.
- It removes many chemicals and drugs from the blood and excretes them in the urine.
- It helps in maintaining the pH of the body fluids.
- It helps in regulating blood pressure by secreting the enzyme renin which activates the renin-angiotensin-aldosterone pathway. Increased renin secretion causes increase in blood pressure.
- It produces two hormones,
  - ✓ **Calcitriol:** It is the active form of vitamin-D helps regulates the calcium homeostasis.
  - ✓ **Erythropoietin:** It stimulates the production of red blood cells.
- Kidneys regulate blood volume: The kidneys adjust blood volume by eliminating water in the urine. Increased blood volume increases the blood pressure.

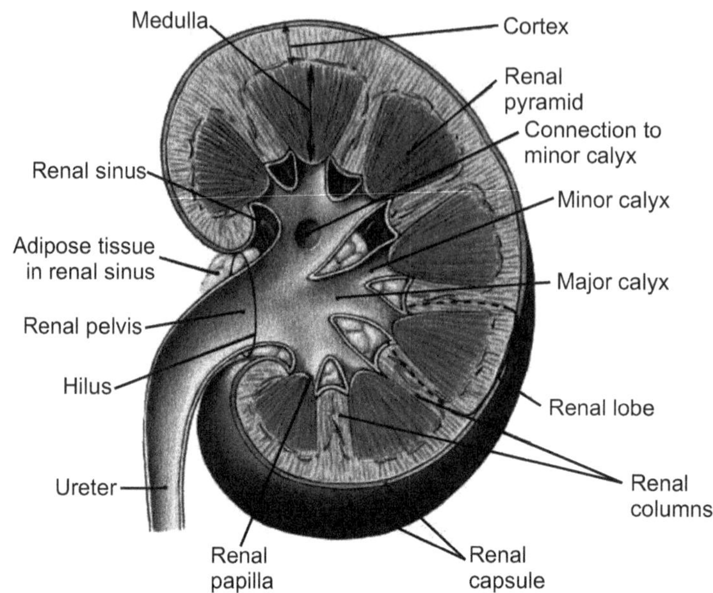

Fig. 5.2: Internal structure of the kidney

5.3 NEPHRONS

- The nephrons are arranged in the renal cortex and renal medulla.
- Morphologically there are two types of nephrons.
  - ✓ **The cortical nephron:** They make up about 80-90% nephrons. They originate in the cortex of the kidney and are more superficial. They extend only a short distance in the medulla.
  - ✓ **The juxtamedullary nephron:** They make up about 10-20% nephrons. These originate at the junction between renal the cortex and the renal medulla and extend deep into the medulla.
- Nephron is the functional unit of the kidneys.
- Each nephron consists of two parts.
  - ✓ **Renal corpuscle:** Where the blood plasma is filtered.
  - ✓ **Renal tubule:** Into which the filtered fluid passes.
- Two components of renal corpuscle are:
- ✓ **Glomerulus (Capillary network)**
- ✓ **Glomerular capsule (Bowman's capsule):** A double walled epithelial cup that surrounds the glomerular capillaries.
- Blood plasma is first filtered in the glomerular capsule and then the filtered fluid passes into the renal tubule which has three parts namely:
  - ✓ Proximal convoluted tubule (PCT)
  - ✓ Loop of Henle (Nephron Loop)
  - ✓ Distal convoluted tubule (DCT)
- The renal corpuscle and both the convoluted tubules lie within the renal cortex, whereas the loop of Henle extends into the renal medulla, makes a hairpin turn and then returns to the renal cortex.

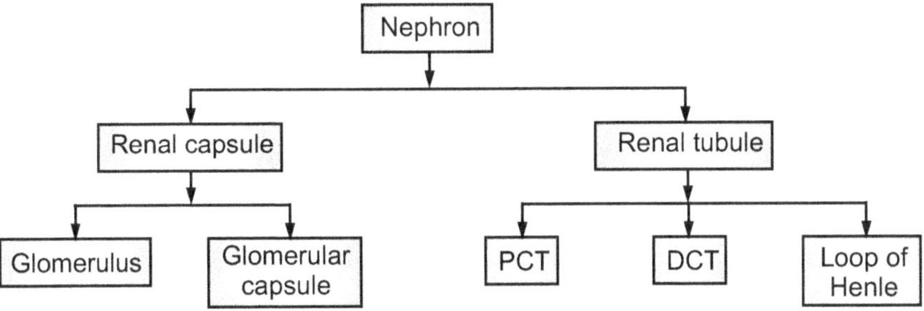

Fig. 5.3: Classification of nephron

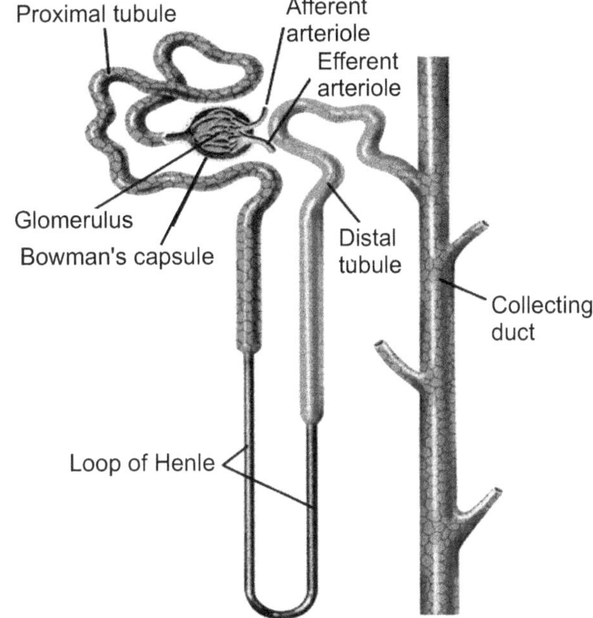

Fig. 5.4: Nephron

Renal Corpuscle

- It has two components.
  - ✓ **Glomerulus:** A tuft of capillary loops called as glomerulus.
  - ✓ **Glomerular (Bowman's) capsule:** It is surrounded by a double walled epithelial cup called as glomerular capsule.
- The blood enters a glomerulus through afferent arteriole and exits through an efferent arteriole.
- The outer wall or parietal layer of the glomerular capsule is separated from the inner wall known as visceral layer by the capsular space.
- As blood flows through the glomerular capillaries, water and other solutes filter from blood plasma into the capsular space.
- Large plasma proteins and formed elements in blood do not normally pass through.
- From the capsular space, the filtered fluid passes into the renal tubule.

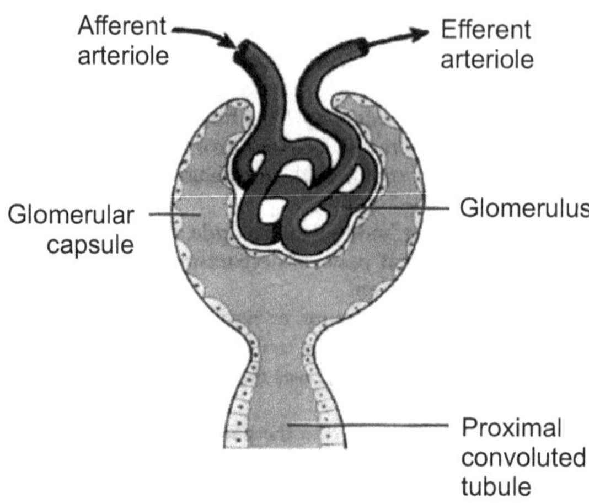

Fig. 5.5: Glomerular (Bowman's) capsule

Renal Tubule

The renal tubule consists of:

- **Proximal convoluted tubule (PCT):** It starts from the Bowman's capsule. It is made up of simple cuboidal epithelium having microvilli forming the brush border on the inner side of tubule. This increases the internal surface area which helps the PCT to reabsorb the fluid. PCT continues with the descending loop of Henle.

- **Loop of Henle:** It is made up of the ascending limb and descending limb. These limbs are thin walled and form a sharp hairpin like structure. The loop of Henle is longer and deeper. The ascending limb becomes wide and thick towards the cortex.

- **Distal convoluted tubule (DCT):** It is a highly coiled structure starting from the ascending limb of loop of Henle. The internal surface of DCT is lined by cuboidal epithelium.

- **Collecting Duct:** The distal convoluted tubule continues with the collecting ducts. The cells of the collecting tubules are highly columnar.

5.4 PHYSIOLOGY OF URINE FORMATION

- The kidneys form the urine which passes through the ureter to the bladder for temporary storage.

- Three main processes involved in the formation of urine.
  - ✓ Glomerular filtration
  - ✓ Selective reabsorption
  - ✓ Tubular secretion

Glomerular Filtration

- The first step in production of urine is called as glomerular filtration.

- The principle of filtration is forcing of fluids and dissolved substances through a membrane by pressure.

- It occurs in the renal corpuscle of kidneys across the endothelial-capsular membrane.

- Blood pressure forces water and dissolved blood components through the endothelial-capsular membrane.
- The resulting fluid is called as filtrate.
- The filtrate contains all the materials present in the blood except the formed elements and large plasma proteins that cannot pass through the endothelial-capsular membrane.

Structures that enhance the blood-filtering capacity of the renal corpuscles

1. **Glomerular capillaries are long:** The glomerular capillaries are very long and present a large surface area for filtration.
2. **The filter (endothelial-capsular membrane) is porous and thin:** The endothelial-capsular membrane is very thin 0.1 um and porous. Water, glucose, vitamins, amino acids, small proteins, nitrogenous waste and ions easily pass into the capsular space.
3. **Capillary blood pressure is high:** The efferent arteriole is smaller in diameter than the afferent arteriole. Thus, blood pressure is higher in the glomerular capillaries than in capillaries elsewhere in the body. A higher blood pressure means more filtration.

Net Filtration Pressure (NFP)

- In the glomerulus, blood filtration depends on three main processes.
  - ✓ **Glomerulus blood hydrostatic pressure (60 mm Hg)**
- This pressure favours filtration. It is the pressure exerted by blood on the walls of the capillaries (60 mm Hg). Two other forces that oppose glomerular blood hydrostatic pressure are the capsular hydrostatic pressure and blood osmotic pressure.
  - ✓ **Capsular hydrostatic pressure (15 mm Hg)**
- As the fluid enters the capsular space, it is opposed by the walls of the capsule as well as the fluid already present in the capsular space. As a result, some of the filtrate is pushed back into the capillary.
  - ✓ **Blood osmotic pressure (27 mm Hg)**
- The second force opposing filtration process is the blood osmotic pressure which is due to the presence of proteins in the blood plasma. As the protein concentration is very high as compared to that of the glomerular filtrate, some water moves back from the filtrate to the glomerular capillaries.
- NFP = Glomerular blood hydrostatic pressure – (Capsular hydrostatic pressure + Blood colloid osmotic pressure)
- NFP = (60 mm Hg) – (15 mm Hg + 27 mm Hg)

  = 60 – 42

  = 18 mm Hg

- This means that, a pressure of about 18 mm Hg causes normal amount of plasma (minus plasma proteins) to filter from the glomerulus into the capsular space.

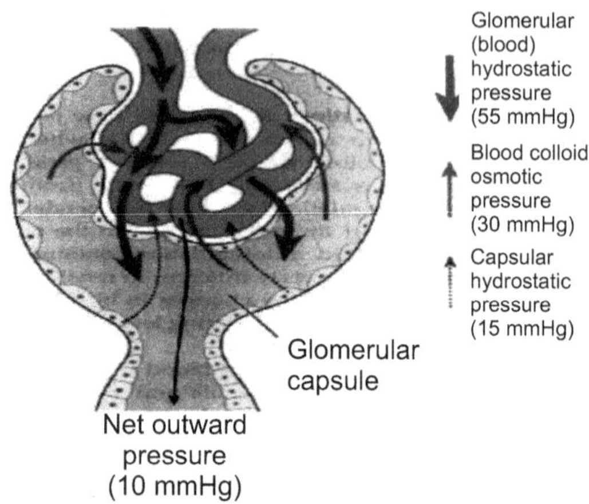

Fig. 5.6: Net filtration pressure

Glomerular Filtration Rate (GFR)

- The amount of filtrate that forms in all the renal corpuscles of both kidneys every minute is called as glomerular filtration rate.
- In a normal adult, GFR is 125 ml/min-about 180 litres a day.

Tubular Reabsorption

- As the fluid passes through the renal tubules, about 99% of it is reabsorbed and returned to the blood.
- Thus, only 1% of the filtrate leaves the body as urine (about 1.5 litres/day).
- The movement of water and solutes back into the blood of a peritubular capillary called as tubular reabsorption.
- The solutes are reabsorbed both by active and passive processes.
- Solutes that are reabsorbed includes glucose, amino acids, urea and ions such as Na^+, K^+, Ca^{+2}, Cl^-, HCO_3^- and HPO_4^-
- Water reabsorption occurs by the passive process of osmosis.
- Reabsorption is regulated by various hormones.
    - ✓ **Parathyroid hormone:** It is secreted by the parathyroid gland and together with calcitonin from the thyroid gland regulates the reabsorption of calcium and phosphate ions.
    - ✓ **Antidiuretic hormone:** It is secreted by the posterior lobe of the pituitary gland. It increases the water reabsorption.
    - ✓ **Aldosterone:** It is secreted by the adrenal cortex. It increases the reabsorption of sodium ions and excretion of potassium ions.
    - ✓ **Atrial natriuretic hormone (ANP):** It is secreted by the atria of the heart. It decreases the reabsorption of sodium ions and water in PCT and collecting ducts. It also inhibits the secretion of anti-diuretic hormone and aldosterone.

Tubular Secretion

- The third process involved in urine formation is the tubular secretion.
- Tubular reabsorption returns substances from the filtrate into the blood; tubular secretion removes materials from the blood and adds them to the filtrate.
- These secreted substances are potassium ions, hydrogen ions, ammonium ions, creatinine and drugs like penicillin and para-aminohippuric acid.
- Tubular secretions of hydrogen ions are important in normal blood pH maintenance.

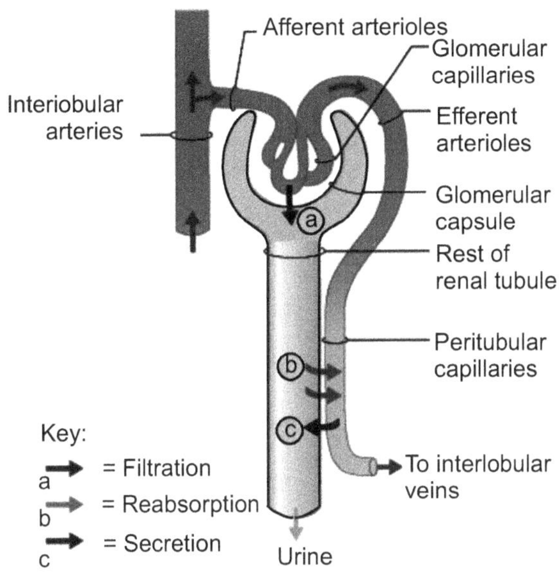

Fig. 5.7: Urine formation process

5.5 COMPOSITION OF URINE

- **Colour:** Yellow/amber coloured
- **Specific gravity:** 1.003 to 1.030
- **pH:** 6
- **Volume:** 1 to 2 litres/day
- **Odour:** Aromatic and become ammonia like on standing
- **Composition:** Water (96%), urea (2%), uric acid, creatinine, ammonia, sodium, potassium, chlorides, phosphates, sulphates and oxalates (2%).
- Urine production is decreased during the sleep and exercise.

5.6 URETER

- There are two ureters - one for each kidney.
- These are the tubes that convey urine from the kidneys to the urinary bladder.
- They are 25 to 30 cm long and 3 mm thick.

- The ureter is continuous with the funnel shaped renal pelvis.
- It passes downwards through the abdominal cavity, behind the peritoneum and passes obliquely through the posterior wall of the bladder.
- Because of this arrangement, when urine accumulates and the pressure in the bladder rises, the ureters are compressed and the openings occluded.
- **Histology:** Ureters consist of three coats of tissue.
- **Inner layer (Mucosa):** It is made up of transitional epithelium tissue.
- **Middle layer (Muscular layer):** It is made up of smooth muscles tissue.
- **Outer layer (Fibrous tissue):** It is made up of fibrous connective tissue
- The function of ureter is transportation of urine from renal pelvis to the urinary bladder.

5.7 URINARY BLADDER

- The urinary bladder is a pear-shaped organ, but becomes more oval as it fills with urine.
- It acts as a temporary reservoir for urine.
- It lies in the pelvic cavity and its size and position vary depending upon the amount of urine it contains.
- When distended, the bladder rises into the abdominal cavity.
- The bladder capacity is smaller in female because the uterus occupies the space just above the bladder.
- It is divided into two parts.
  - ✓ Body
  - ✓ Neck
- Neck is the funnel shaped extension of body; it connects with the urethra and is 2-3 cm long.
- When empty, the urinary bladder is tetrahedral and lies within the pelvis.
- When filled with urine it is oval and extends into the abdominal cavity.
- The three orifices in the bladder wall form a triangle or trigone.
- The upper two orifices of the ureters and lower orifice of urethra form the trigone.
- The internal urethral sphincters in the upper part of the urethra control the outflow of urine from the bladder.
- **Histology:** The urinary bladder is made up of three layers. Namely;
  - ✓ Inner layer (Mucosa): It is made up of transitional epithelium tissue.
  - ✓ Middle layer (Muscular layer): It is made up of smooth muscles tissue.
  - ✓ Outer layer (Fibrous tissue): It is made up of fibrous connective tissue.

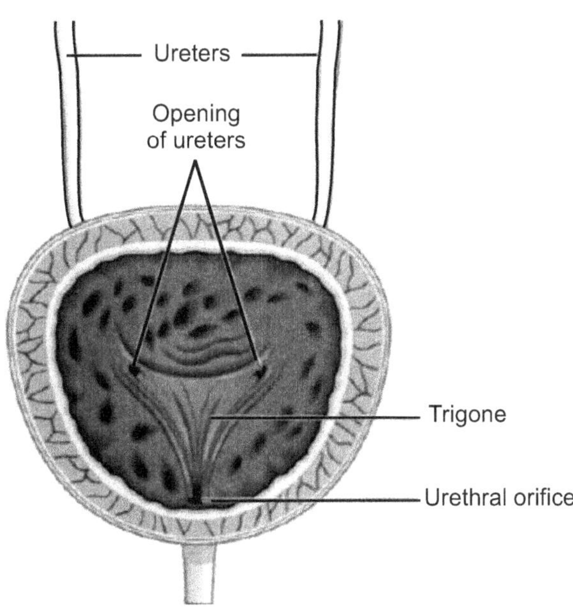

Fig. 5.8: Urinary Bladder

5.8 URETHRA

- It is a small tube leading from the floor of the urinary bladder to the exterior of the body.
- It is longer in males than in females.
- Male: It is 20 cm long.
- Female: It is 4 cm long.
- Wall of the female urethra consists of three coats.
  - ✓ **Inner layer (Mucosa):** It is made up of transitional epithelium tissue.
  - ✓ **Middle layer (Submucosa):** It is made up of spongy tissue coat.
  - ✓ **Outer layer (Muscular layer):** It is made up of stratified squamous tissue.
- Male urethra is divided into 3 parts.
  - ✓ Prostatic urethra: It is 3 cm long
  - ✓ Membranous urethra: It is 1.5 to 2 cm long.
  - ✓ Spongy urethra: It is 15 cm long (penile part).

5.9 RENIN-ANGIOTENSIN-ALDOSTERONE SYSTEM (RAA)

- Renin-angiotensin-aldosterone is a hormone system that regulates the blood pressure and the water (fluid) balance.
1. Stimuli that initiate the renin–angiotensin–aldosterone pathway include dehydration, Na^+ deficiency or haemorrhage.
2. These conditions cause a decrease in the blood volume.
3. Decreased the blood volume leads to decreased blood pressure.
4. Lowered blood pressure stimulates the juxtaglomerular cells of the kidney, to secrete the enzyme renin.

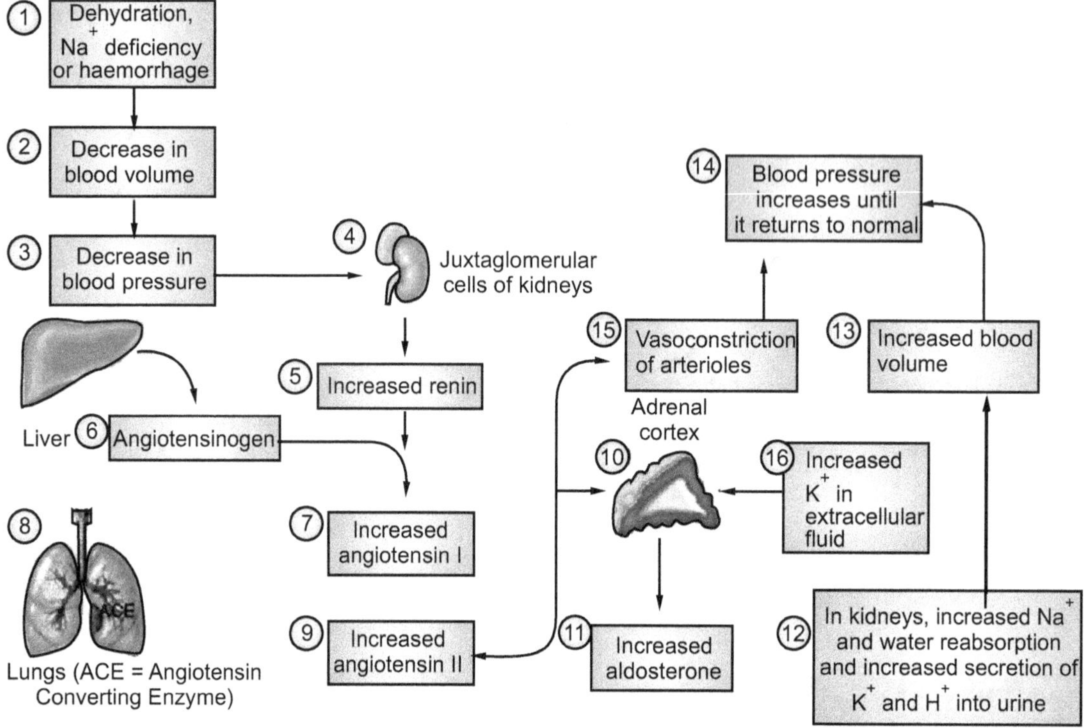

Fig. 5.9: Renin-angiotensin-aldosterone system

5. The level of renin in the blood increases.

6. Renin converts angiotensinogen, a plasma protein produced by the liver, into angiotensin-I.

7. Blood containing increased levels of angiotensin I circulates in the body.

8. Angiotensin-converting enzyme (ACE) in the lungs converts angiotensin I into angiotensin-II hormone.

9. The blood level of angiotensin II increases

10. Angiotensin II stimulates the adrenal cortex to secrete aldosterone.

11. The blood containing increased levels of aldosterone circulates to the kidneys.

12. In the kidneys, aldosterone increases reabsorption of sodium ions and water and increases secretion of potassium ions and hydrogen ions into the urine.

13. With increased water reabsorption by the kidneys, blood volume increases.

14. As blood volume increases, blood pressure increases to normal.

15. Angiotensin-II also stimulates the contraction of smooth muscle in the walls of arterioles. The resulting vasoconstriction of the arterioles increases the blood pressure.

16. Besides angiotensin II, a second stimulator of aldosterone secretion is an increase in the potassium ion concentration of blood. A decrease in the blood potassium ion level has the opposite effect.

5.10 ACID-BASE BALANCE

- In order to maintain the normal pH of blood, the cells of the proximal convoluted tubules secrete hydrogen ions.
- In the filtrate they combine with buffers as shown below:
    - ✓ Hydrogen ions + Bicarbonate = Carbonic acid ($H^+ + HCO_3^- \longrightarrow H_2CO_3$)
    - ✓ Hydrogen ions + Ammonia = Ammonium ions ($H^+ + NH_3 \longrightarrow NH_4^+$)
    - ✓ Hydrogen ions + Hydrogen phosphate = Dihydrogen phosphate
    $$(H^+ + HPO_3^{2-} \longrightarrow H_2PO_3^-)$$
    - ✓ Carbonic acid is converted to carbon dioxide (CO_2) and water (H_2O), and the CO_2 is reabsorbed maintaining the buffering capacity of the blood.
- Hydrogen ions are excreted in the urine as ammonium salts and hydrogen phosphate.
- The normal pH of urine varies from 4.5 to 8 depending on diet, time and a variety of other factors.

5.11 ELECTROLYTE BALANCE

- The changes in the electrolytes concentration of body fluids may occurs due to the changes in
    - ✓ The body water content or
    - ✓ The electrolyte levels
- There are several mechanisms that maintain the balance between water and electrolyte concentration.

Sodium and Potassium balance

- Sodium is the positively charged cation in the extracellular fluid and potassium is the most common positively charged intracellular cation.
- Sodium is a constituent of almost all foods and it is often added to the food during cooking.
- It is excreted mainly in the urine and the sweat.
- Sodium is the normal constituent of urine and the amount excreted is regulated by the aldosterone hormone, secreted by the adrenal cortex.
- The cells in the afferent arteriole of the nephron are stimulated to produce renin enzyme by sympathetic stimulation, low blood volume or by low blood pressure.
- Renin converts the plasma angiotensinogen, produced by the liver, to angiotensin-I.
- Angiotensin converting enzyme (ACE), formed in the lungs converts angiotensin-I into angiotensin-II which is a potent vasoconstrictor and increases the blood pressure.
- Renin and raised blood potassium levels also stimulate the adrenal gland to secrete aldosterone.
- Water is reabsorbed with sodium and together they increase the blood volume, leading to reduced renin secretion through the negative feedback mechanism.
- When sodium reabsorption is increased, potassium excretion is increased, indirectly reducing intracellular potassium ion concentration.

- The amount of sodium excreted in the sweat is insignificant except when sweating is excessive.
- Normally, the renal mechanism maintains the concentration of sodium and potassium ions within physiological limits.
- Sodium and potassium occur in high concentrations in digestive juices - sodium in gastric juice and potassium in pancreatic and intestinal juice.
- Normally these ions are reabsorbed by the colon but following acute and prolonged diarrhoea they may be excreted in large quantities with resultant electrolyte imbalance.

Calcium balance

- Regulation of calcium levels is achieved by the secretion of parathyroid hormone and calcitonin.
- The distal collecting tubule reabsorbs more calcium in response to parathyroid hormone secretion and reabsorbs less calcium in response to secretion to calcitonin.

5.12 WATER BALANCE

- The source of body water is dietary food and fluid and small amount is formed by the metabolic processes.
- Water is excreted in expired air, as a constituent of the faeces, through the skin as sweat and as the main constituent of the urine.
- The amount lost in the expired air and in the faeces is fairly constant and the amount of sweat produced is associated with the maintenance of normal body temperature.
- The balance between fluid intake and output is controlled by the kidneys.
- The minimum urinary output is about 500 ml per day.
- The amount produced in excess is controlled by antidiuretic hormone (ADH) released into the blood by the posterior lobe of the pituitary gland.

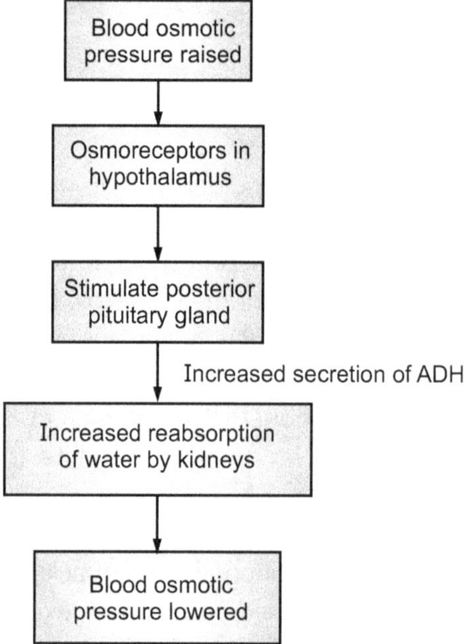

Fig. 5.10: Maintenance of water balance

- Sensory nerve cells in the hypothalamus (osmoreceptors) detect changes in the osmotic pressure of the blood.
- Nerve impulses from the osmoreceptors stimulate the posterior lobe of the pituitary gland to release ADH.
- When the osmotic pressure is raised, ADH output is increased and as a result, water reabsorption by the cells in distal convoluted tubules and collecting ducts is increased, reducing the blood osmotic pressure and ADH output.
- When blood volume is increased, stretch receptors in the atria of the heart release atrial natriuretic peptide hormone (ANP).
- This reduces reabsorption of sodium and water by PCT and collecting ducts, meaning that are more sodium and water are excreted.
- This in turn, reduces the blood volume.

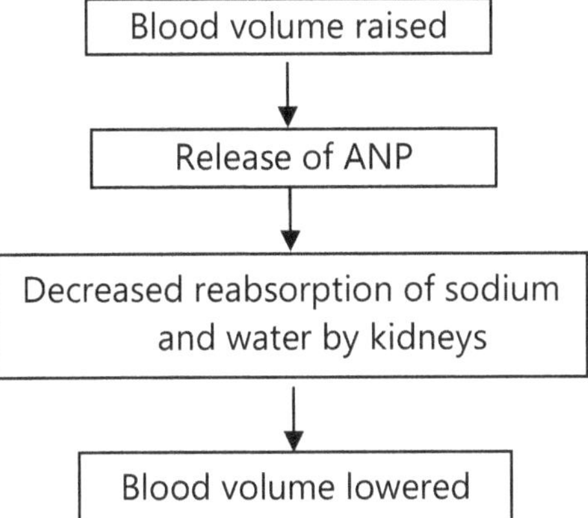

Fig. 5.11: Maintenance of water balance

5.13 RENAL CLEARANCE TEST

- Assessment of kidney function involves evaluation of both the quantity and quality of urine and the amount of wastes substances in the blood.
- The various test are:
  - ✓ Urinalysis
  - ✓ Blood tests
  - ✓ Renal plasma clearance

Urinalysis

- An analysis of the volume, physical, chemical and microscopic properties of the urine is called as urinalysis.

Characteristic of normal urine

- **Volume:** One to two litres in 24 hours.
- **Colour:** Yellow or amber colour but varies with urine concentration and diet. Colour is due to urochrome (pigment produced due to breakdown of bile) and urobilin (due to breakdown of haemoglobin). Concentrated urine is darker in colour.

- **Turbidity:** Transparent when freshly voided but becomes turbid on standing.
- **Odour:** Mildly aromatic but becomes ammonia-like on standing.
- **pH:** Ranges between 4.6 and 8.0. High-protein diets increase acidity; vegetarian diets increase alkalinity.
- **Specific gravity:** In urine, it ranges from 1.001 to 1.035.
- **Albumin:** The presence of excessive albumin in the urine is called as albuminuria.
- **Glucose:** The presence of glucose in the urine is called glucosuria.
- **Red blood cells:** The presence of red blood cells in urine is called hematuria.
- **Ketone bodies:** High levels of ketone bodies in urine are termed as ketonuria.
- **Bilirubin:** The presence of excessive bilirubin in urine is called bilirubinuria.
- **Urobilinogen:** The presence of urobilinogen (breakdown product of hemoglobin) in urine is called urobilinogenuria.
- **Microbes:** The number and type of bacteria vary with specific infections in the urinary tract. One of the most common bacteria is *E. coli*. The most common fungus is the yeast *Candida albicans*. The most frequent protozoan seen is *Trichomonas vaginalis*.

Blood Tests

- Two blood-screening tests can provide information about the kidney function.
  - ✓ Blood urea nitrogen test
  - ✓ Measurement of plasma creatinine

Blood urea nitrogen (BUN) test

- It measures the blood nitrogen that is part of the urea resulting from catabolism and deamination of amino acids.
- When the glomerular filtration rate decreases, BUN rises steeply.
- Normal range for blood urea nitrogen is 5 to 20 mg/dl.

Plasma creatinine test

- It measures the plasma creatinine, which results from the catabolism of creatinine phosphate in the skeletal muscle.
- A creatinine level above 1.5 mg/dL usually is an indication of poor renal function.

Renal plasma clearance

- Renal plasma clearance is an evaluation of how effectively kidneys are removing a given substance from the blood plasma.
- Renal plasma clearance is the volume of blood that is cleared of a substance per unit of time.
- It is usually expressed in millilitres per minute.
- High renal plasma clearance indicates efficient excretion of a substance in the urine; low clearance indicates inefficient excretion.
- Renal plasma clearance of substance $(S) = U \times V/P$
  Where;
  U: Concentration of the substance in urine
  P: Concentration of the substance in plasma
  V: Urine flow rate in ml/min.

5.14 PHYSIOLOGY OF MICTURITION REFLEX

- The urinary bladder acts as a reservoir of urine.
- When 300 to 400 ml of urine has accumulated, afferent autonomic nerve fibres in the bladder wall get stimulated.
- Micturition occurs when autonomic efferent fibres convey impulses to the bladder causing contraction of the detrusor muscle and relaxation of the internal urethral sphincter.
- When the nervous system is fully developed, the micturition reflex is stimulated but sensory impulses pass upwards to the brain and there is an awareness of the desire to pass urine.
- By conscious effort, reflex contraction of the bladder wall and relaxation of the internal sphincter can be inhibited for a limited period of time.
- In adults, micturition occurs when the detrusor muscle contracts and there is reflex relaxation of the internal sphincter and voluntary relaxation of the external sphincter.
- It can be assisted by increasing the pressure within the pelvic cavity, achieved by lowering the diaphragm and contracting the abdominal muscles.
- Over-distension of the bladder is extremely painful, and when this stage is reached there is a tendency for involuntary relaxation of the external sphincter to occur and a small amount of urine to escape, provided there is no mechanical obstruction.

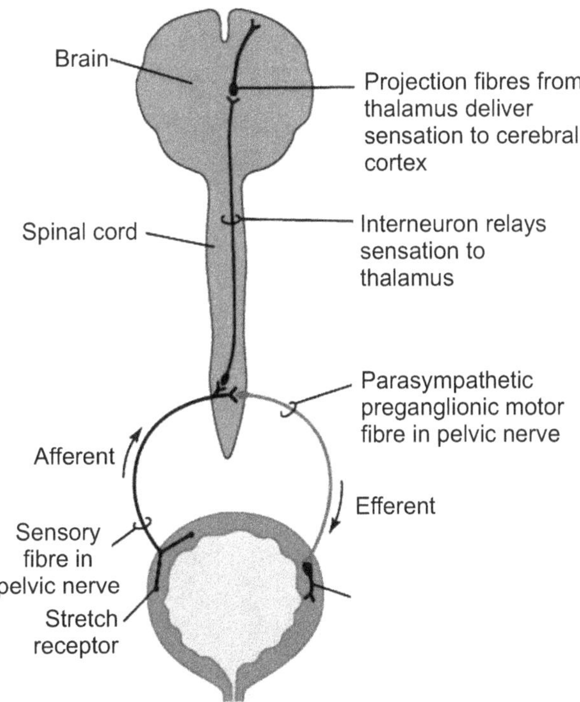

Fig. 5.12: Micturition reflex

5.15 DISORDERS OF THE URINARY SYSTEM

Renal Calculi

- The crystals of salts present in the urine occasionally precipitate and solidify into insoluble stones called as renal calculi or renal stones.
- The commonly found crystals are calcium oxalates, uric acid or calcium phosphate.
- The conditions leading to calculus formation include the ingestion of excessive calcium, low water intake, abnormally alkaline or acidic urine and overactivity of the parathyroid glands.

Urinary tract infection (UTI)

- It is used to describe either an infection of a part of urinary system or the presence of large number of microbes in urine.
- UTI is more common in females because of short length of the urethra.
- The symptom includes painful or burning urination, urgent and frequent urination, low back pain and bed-wetting.
- UTI includes:
  - ✓ **Urethritis:** Inflammation of the urethra
  - ✓ **Cystitis:** Inflammation of the urinary bladder
  - ✓ **Pyelonephritis:** Inflammation of the kidneys

Glomerulonephritis

- It is an inflammation of the kidney that involves the glomeruli.
- The glomeruli become inflamed, swollen and enlarged with blood as the filtration membrane allows blood cells and plasma proteins to enter the filtrate under the diseased condition.
- As a result, the urine contains many red blood cells and lots of protein.
- This inflammation typically results in one or both of the nephrotic or nephritic syndromes.

Nephrotic syndrome

- It is a condition characterised by protein in the urine and hyperlipidaemia (high blood levels of cholesterol, phospholipids and triglycerides).
- The proteinuria is due to an increased permeability of the filtration membrane, which permits proteins, especially albumin, to escape from blood into urine.
- Loss of albumin results in hypoalbuminemia (low blood albumin level) once liver production of albumin fails to meet increased urinary losses.
- Edema, usually seen around the eyes, ankles, feet, and abdomen, occurs in nephrotic syndrome because of loss of albumin from the blood decreases.

Renal failure

- It is a decrease in the glomerular filtration rate.
- There are two types of renal failure:
  - ✓ Acute renal failure (ARF)
  - ✓ Chronic renal failure (CRF)

Acute renal failure

- ✓ The kidneys abruptly stop working entirely.
- ✓ The main feature of ARF is the suppression of urine flow, usually characterised either by oliguria (daily urine output between 50-250 ml) or by anuria (daily urine output less than 50 ml).

Chronic renal failure

- ✓ It refers to a progressive and usually irreversible decline in the glomerular filtration rate.
- ✓ It may result from chronic glomerulonephritis, pyelonephritis, polycystic kidney disease or traumatic loss of kidney tissue.

Polycystic kidney disease (PKD)

- It is most common inherited disorders.
- In PKD, the kidney tubules become riddled with hundreds or thousands of cysts (fluid-filled cavities).
- The cysts are numerous and are fluid-filled, resulting in massive enlargement of the kidneys.
- There are two types of PKD:
    - Autosomal dominant polycystic kidney disease (ADPKD): It is more common.
    - Autosomal recessive polycystic kidney disease (ARPKD): It is less-common.

Urinary bladder cancer

- It is a cancer of the urinary bladder.
- Bladder cancer is one of the common cancers affecting both men and women.
- The most common symptom is bleeding in the urine (hematuria).
- Cigarette smoking is the most significant risk factor with smokers three to four times more likely to suffer from the disease than non-smokers.
- Bladder cancer can be subdivided into superficial and muscle invasive, with the former having much better treatment outcomes than the latter.

QUESTIONS

Short Answer Questions:

1. Enlist the different parts of the urinary system.
2. Draw a neat labelled diagram of the urinary system.
3. Draw a neat labelled diagram of the nephron.
4. Give the composition of urine.
5. Write a note on nephron.
6. Write a note on the renin angiotensin aldosterone system.
7. Explain the internal structure of kidney.
8. Write a note on micturition process.
9. Explain the urine formation process.
10. Explain the electrolyte balance.
11. What is net filtration pressure (NFP)?

Long Answer Questions:

1. Describe the different renal clearance tests.
2. Explain the physiology of urine formation.
3. Draw a neat labeled diagram of L.S. of kidney. Explain functions of the kidney in detail.
4. Draw a neat labeled diagram of the nephron and explain in detail the physiology of urine formation.

UNIT V

Chapter 6...

ENDOCRINE SYSTEM

♦ LEARNING OBJECTIVES ♦

❖ To distinguish between exocrine and endocrine glands.

❖ To describe types and functions of hormones.

❖ To describe the general mechanisms of hormone action.

❖ To describe the location, histology, hormones, and functions of the anterior and posterior pituitary.

❖ To describe the location, histology, hormones, and functions of the thyroid gland.

❖ To describe the location, histology, hormone, and functions of the parathyroid glands.

❖ To describe the location, histology, hormones, and functions of the adrenal glands.

❖ To describe the location, histology, hormones, and functions of the pancreatic islets.

❖ To describe the location, hormones, and functions of the male and female gonads.

❖ To describe the location, histology, hormone, and functions of the pineal gland.

6.1 INTRODUCTION

The endocrine system is the collection of glands that secrete hormones directly into the circulatory system to be carried to a distant target organ. The major endocrine glands include the pineal gland, pituitary gland, pancreas, ovaries, testes, thyroid gland, parathyroid gland and adrenal glands. Circulating or local hormones of the endocrine system contribute to homeostasis by regulating the activity and growth of target cells in the body. Hormones regulate the metabolism processes of the body.

Endocrinology is the branch of science that deals with the study of structure and function of the endocrine glands, their disorders and their treatment.

6.2 BODY GLANDS

These are divided into two types:

Exocrine Glands

- These are the glands which possess ducts and secrete their secretions through ducts.

- E.g. Salivary gland, sweat glands and sebaceous glands.

(6.1)

Endocrine Glands

* These are the ductless glands and secrete their secretions directly in the surrounding spaces which are further distributed throughout the body by blood.
* E.g. Pituitary gland, thyroid gland, parathyroid gland, adrenal gland and pineal gland
* Several organs and tissues are not endocrine glands but contain cells that secrete hormones.
* E.g. Hypothalamus, thymus, pancreas, ovaries, testes, kidneys, stomach, liver, small intestine, skin, heart, adipose tissue and placenta

6.3 HORMONES

* These are mediator molecules that are released in one part of the body but regulate the activity of cells in other parts of the body.
* Hormones regulate important body processes and functions including growth, reproduction and metabolism.

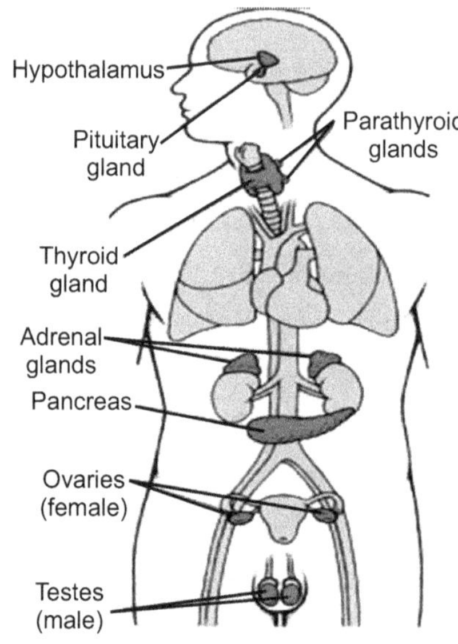

Fig. 6.1: Endocrine system

Types of Hormones

✓ **Circulating hormone:** They pass from the secretory cells into the interstitial fluid and then into the blood.

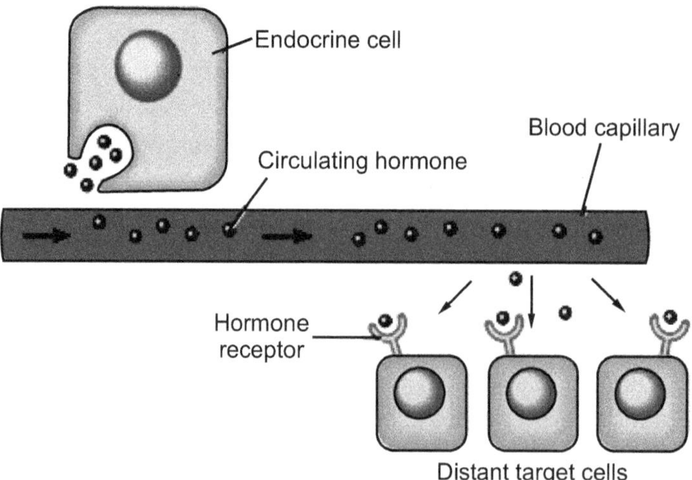

Fig. 6.2: Circulating hormone

- ✓ **Local hormones:** They act locally on neighbouring cells or on the same cell that secrete them without first entering the bloodstream.
- Among local hormones are those that act on neighbouring cells called as paracrine and those that act on the same cell that secrete them called as autocrine.

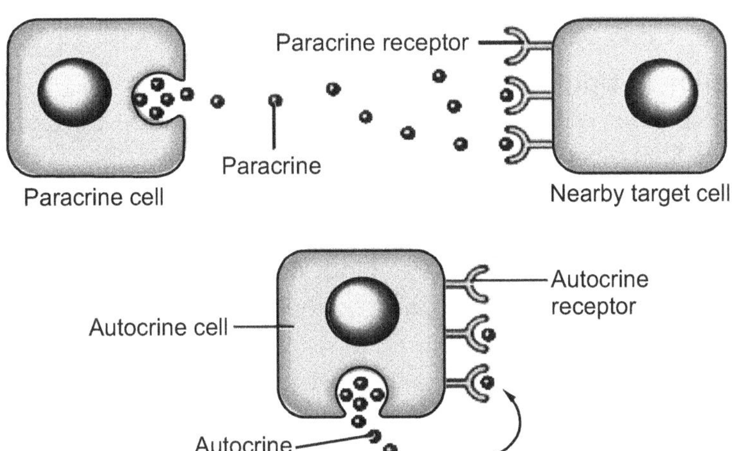

Fig. 6.3: Local hormone

Functions of Hormones

- Control growth and development
- Regulate chemical composition and volume of the internal environment (interstitial fluid)
- Regulate metabolism and energy balance
- Regulate contraction of smooth and cardiac muscle fibres
- Regulate glandular secretions
- Involved in some immune system activities
- Regulate operation of reproductive systems
- Helps establish the circadian rhythms

6.4 CHEMICAL CLASSES OF HORMONES

Hormones are divided into two broad classes:
- ✓ Lipid soluble hormone
- ✓ Water soluble hormone

Lipid Soluble Hormones

- Lipid soluble hormones are fat soluble hormones.
- They affect the cells by binding to receptors of the target cells.
- The structure of lipid soluble hormones is derived from cholesterol.
- They can move through the lipid bilayer as they are lipid soluble.
- These include the steroid hormone and thyroid hormone.

Steroid Hormones

- These are derived from cholesterol and they differ in the ring structure and the side chains attached to it.
- All steroid hormones are lipid soluble.

- E.g. Cortisol and aldosterone produced by the adrenal glands, estrogen and progesterone produced by the ovaries and testosterone produced by the testes.

Thyroid Hormones

- Two thyroid hormones (T_3 and T_4) are synthesised by attaching iodine to amino acid tyrosine.
- The benzene ring of tyrosine plus the attached iodine makes T_3 and T_4 very lipid soluble.

Mechanism of Action of Lipid Soluble Hormone

- A free lipid-soluble hormone molecule diffuses from the blood through interstitial fluid, and through the lipid bilayer of the plasma membrane into a cell.
- The hormone binds to receptor and activates the receptors located within the cytosol or nucleus.
- The activated receptor–hormone complex binds a specific DNA sequence.
- Binding initiates the process of DNA transcription to form mRNA (Double stranded DNA is converted to single stranded mRNA).
- The mRNA leaves the nucleus and enters the cytosol.
- The mRNA directs synthesis of a new protein on the ribosomes.
- The new proteins alter the cell's activity.

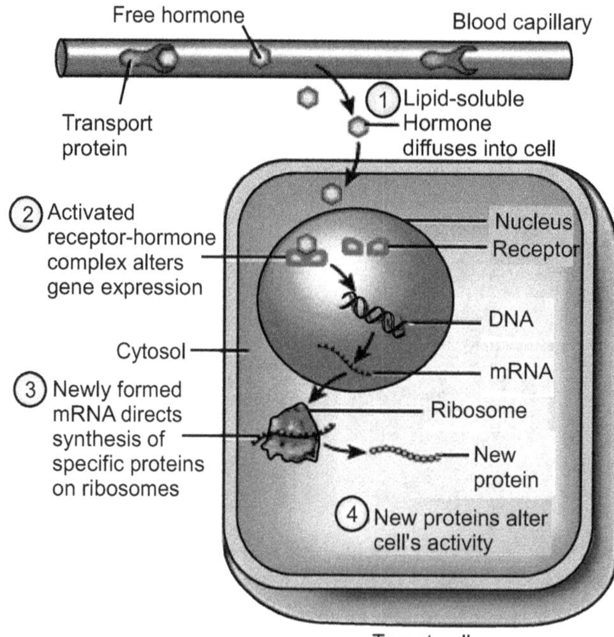

Fig. 6.4: Mechanism of action of lipid soluble hormone

Water Soluble Hormones

- These hormones are soluble in water.
- These hormones cannot pass through the target cell membranes.
- They affect the cells by binding to receptors on the surface of target cell.
- These include the amine hormones, peptide hormones, protein hormones and eicosanoid hormones.

Amine hormones

- These are synthesised by decarboxylating and modifying certain amino acids.
- E.g. Histamine is synthesised from the amino acid histidine by mast cells and platelets.
- Serotonin and melatonin are derived from the amino acid tryptophan.

Peptide and Protein Hormones

- These are polymers of amino acids.
- The smaller peptide hormones consist of a chain of 3 to 49 amino acids.
- Larger protein hormone includes 50 to 200 amino acids.
- E.g. Peptide hormones: Antidiuretic hormones and Oxytocin, Protein hormones: Human growth hormone and insulin

Eicosanoid Hormones

- These are derived from arachidonic acid - a 20 carbon fatty acid.
- There are two major types - prostaglandins and leukotrienes

Mechanism of Action of Water Soluble Hormone

- Amine, peptide, protein and eicosanoid hormones are water-soluble hormones that bind to receptors on the surface of target cell.

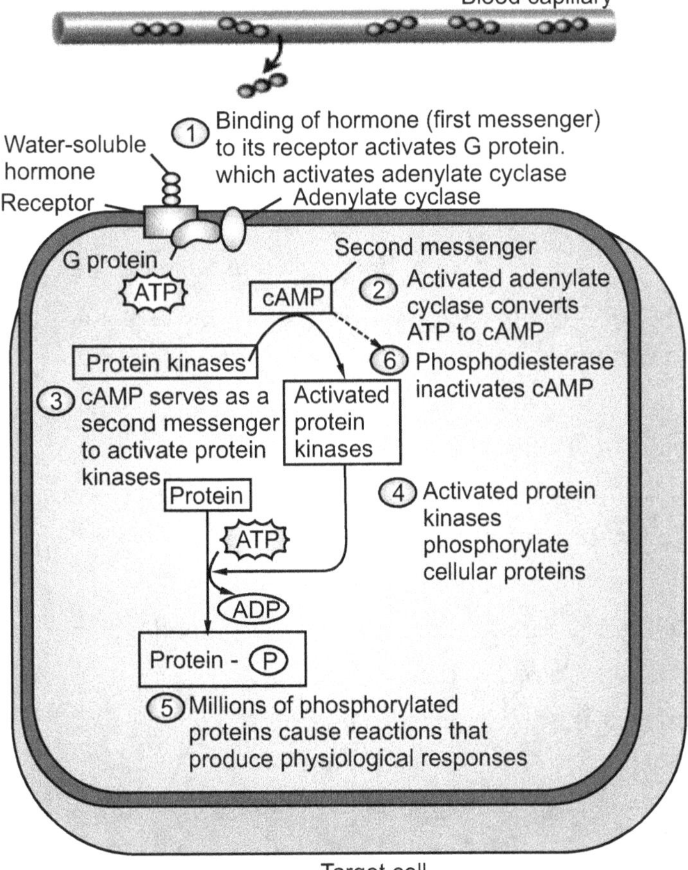

Fig. 6.5: Mechanism of action of water soluble hormone

- When a water soluble hormone binds to its receptor at the outer surface of the plasma membrane, it acts as the first messenger.
- The first messenger (the hormone) causes production of a second messenger cyclic AMP (cAMP) inside the cell, where specific hormone-stimulated responses take place.
- A water-soluble hormone (the first messenger) diffuses from the blood through interstitial fluid and then binds to receptor on the surface of a target cell.
- The hormone–receptor complex activates a membrane protein called a G-protein.
- The activated G protein in turn activates adenylate cyclase.
- Adenylate cyclase converts adenosine triphosphate (ATP) into cyclic AMP.
- Cyclic AMP (the second messenger) activates one or more protein kinases, which may be free in the cytosol or bound to the plasma membrane.
- A protein kinase is an enzyme that phosphorylates the cellular proteins.
- The ATP is then converted into adenosine diphosphate (ADP).
- Activated protein kinases phosphorylate one or more cellular proteins.
- Phosphorylation activates some of these proteins and inactivates others.
- A phosphorylated protein in turn produces the physiological responses.

6.5 HYPOTHALAMUS AND PITUITARY GLAND

- It is a pea-shaped structure that measures 1–1.5 cm in diameter and approximately 1 gm in weight.
- It lies in the bony cavity at the base of brain called as Sella turcica.
- It attaches to the hypothalamus by a stalk called as infundibulum.
- It is divided into two separate parts;
  - ✓ Anterior pituitary (Anterior lobe)/Adenohypophysis
  - ✓ Posterior pituitary (Posterior lobe)/Neurohypophysis

Adenohypophysis: It accounts for about 75% of total weight of gland.

- The anterior pituitary consists of two parts.
  - ✓ The pars distalis: It is the larger portion
  - ✓ The pars tuberalis: It forms a sheath around the infundibulum.

Neurohypophysis: It consists of two parts
  - ✓ The pars nervosa: It is the larger bulbar portion.
  - ✓ The infundibulum

- Pituitary gland is slightly larger in females than in males.
- In females during pregnancy the size increases due to increased secretion of gonadotropin hormone (Follicle Stimulating Hormone and Luteinising Hormone).

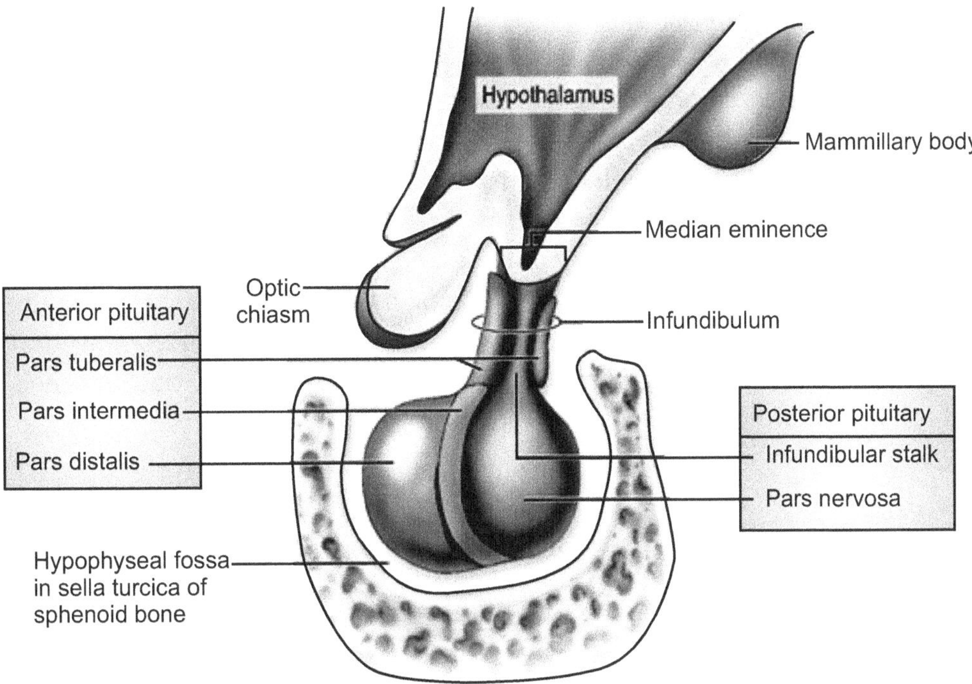

Fig. 6.6: Pituitary gland

Hormones secreted by anterior pituitary

- It makes about 70% of the pituitary gland and is mainly made of five different types of secretory cells.
- These five different types of cells are responsible for production of seven major hormones.
- The five different types of cells are:
  - ✓ Somatotrophs
  - ✓ Thyrotrophs
  - ✓ Gonadotrophs
  - ✓ Lactotrophs
  - ✓ Corticotrophs
- **Somatotrophs:** About 30-40% of the cells of the anterior pituitary gland are somatotrophs. These cells are responsible for secretion of human growth hormone that stimulate general body growth and regulate aspects of metabolism.
- **Thyrotrophs:** About 5% of the cells of the anterior pituitary glands are thyrotrophs. These are responsible for secretion of thyroid stimulating hormone that controls the activities of the thyroid gland.
- **Gonadotrophs:** About 4-5% of the cells of the anterior pituitary gland are gonadotrophs. They secrete two powerful hormones that are responsible for controlling sexual development and function.
  - ✓ Follicle stimulating hormone (FSH)
  - ✓ Luteinizing hormone (LH)

- They stimulate secretion of estrogen and progesterone and maturation of oocytes in the ovaries.
- They stimulate sperm production and secretion of testosterone in the testes.
- **Lactotrophs:** About 3 to 5% of the cells of the anterior pituitary gland are lactotrophs. They secrete prolactin which initiates milk production in the mammary gland.
- **Corticotrophs:** About 20 % of the cells of the anterior pituitary gland are corticotrophs. They secrete two different types of hormones.
  - ✓ Adrenocorticotropin hormone (ACTH): Stimulates the adrenal cortex to secrete glucocorticoids such as Cortisol.
  - ✓ Melanocyte stimulating hormone (MSH): Stimulates the production and release of melanin by melanocytes in skin and hair.

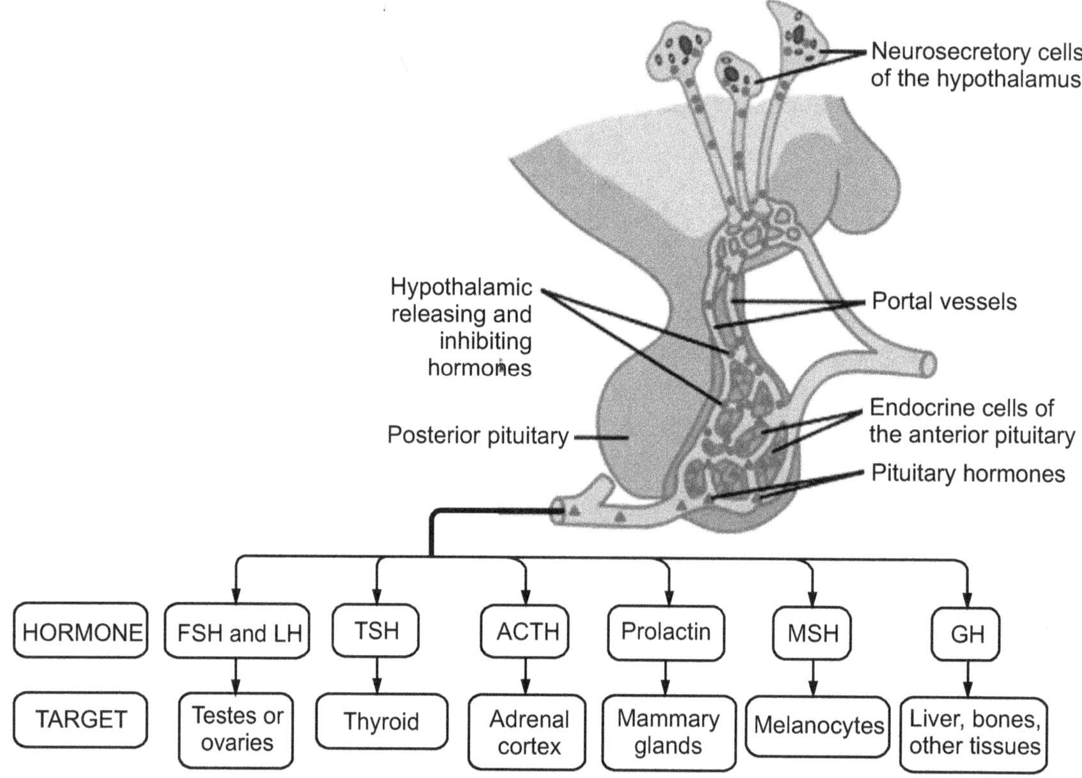

Fig. 6.7: Hormones secreted by anterior pituitary gland

Human Growth Hormone (hGH)

- Somatotrophs are the most numerous cells in the anterior pituitary.
- Somatotrophs secretes the human growth hormone which is the most abundant anterior pituitary hormone.
- Human growth hormone is also known as somatotropin or somatropin. It stimulates growth, cell reproduction, regeneration and regulates metabolism.
- Its secretion is controlled by the hypothalamus through release of growth releasing hormone and growth inhibiting hormone.

- This hormone promotes the growth of the body cells and is involved in protein anabolism, tissue repair, lipolysis and elevation of blood glucose concentration.

Thyroid Stimulating Hormone (TSH)

- Thyroid-stimulating hormone stimulates the synthesis and secretion of the two thyroid hormones, tri-iodothyronine (T_3) and thyroxine (T_4) produced by the thyroid gland.
- Thyrotropin-releasing hormone (TRH) from the hypothalamus controls TSH secretion.
- TRH triggers the pituitary gland to release TSH.
- TSH levels rise and fall in response to changes in the concentration of free thyroxin (T4).
- TSH is elevated if the thyroid gland is not producing adequate thyroid hormone, and suppressed if it is producing excess thyroid hormone.

Follicle Stimulating Hormone (FSH)

- The gonadotrophs are responsible for secreting two powerful hormones which control sexual function.
- These hormones are;
  - ✓ Follicle stimulating hormones (FSH)
  - ✓ Luteinizing hormones (LH)
- In females, ovaries are the target organs for the secretion of FSH.
- FSH initiates the development of several ovarian follicles which are saclike arrangement of secretory cells that surrounds developing oocytes.
- FSH also stimulates follicular cells to secrete estrogens (female sex hormone).
- In males, FSH stimulates sperm production in the testes.
- Gonadotropin releasing hormone (GnRH) from the hypothalamus stimulates FSH release.
- In female, LH triggers ovulation - the release of secondary oocytes (future ovum) by an ovary.
- LH stimulates the formation of corpus luteum (structure formed after ovulation) in the ovary and secretion of progesterone (another female sex hormone) by corpus luteum.
- Together FSH and LH also stimulate the secretion of estrogen by the ovarian cells.
- Estrogen and progesterone prepare the uterus for implantation of fertilised ovum and help prepare the mammary gland for milk production.
- In males, LH stimulates cells in the testes to secrete testosterone.

Prolactin (PRL)

- Prolactin together with other hormones initiates and maintains milk secretion by the mammary glands and promotes the development of breast.
- This hormone stimulates lactation (milk production) and has a direct effect on the breasts immediately after parturition (childbirth).
- Ejection of milk from the mammary glands depends on the hormone oxytocin, which is released from the posterior pituitary.
- The blood level of prolactin is stimulated by prolactin releasing hormone (PRH) released from the hypothalamus and it is lowered by prolactin inhibiting hormone (PIH, dopamine) and by an increased blood level of prolactin.
- Breast tenderness just before the menstruation may be caused by elevated prolactin level.

Melanocyte Stimulating Hormone (MSH)

- Melanocyte-stimulating hormone increases skin pigmentation by stimulating the dispersion of melanin granules in the melanocytes.
- Excessive levels of corticotropin-releasing hormone (CRH) can stimulate MSH release.
- Dopamine inhibits the MSH release.
- The hypothalamus secretes both inhibitory and excitatory hormones that regulate the secretion of melanocyte stimulating hormone.

Adrenocorticotropic Hormone (ACTH)

- ACTH is secreted from the anterior pituitary in response to corticotropin-releasing hormone from the hypothalamus.
- Adrenocorticotropic hormone stimulates and regulates the activity of the adrenal cortex.
- The adrenal glands in turn make a hormone called as cortisol which helps the body to manage stress.
- When cortisol levels rise, ACTH levels normally fall.
- When cortisol levels fall, ACTH levels normally rise.

Hormones Secreted by Posterior Pituitary

- Posterior pituitary does not synthesise hormones but it stores and releases two hormones which are synthesised by the hypothalamus.
- It consists of axons and axon terminals of more than 10,000 neurosecretory cells.
- The axon terminals in the posterior pituitary are associated with specialised neuroglia called pituicytes.
- These two major hormones are:
    - ✓ Oxytocin
    - ✓ Antidiuretic hormone (ADH) or Vasopressin

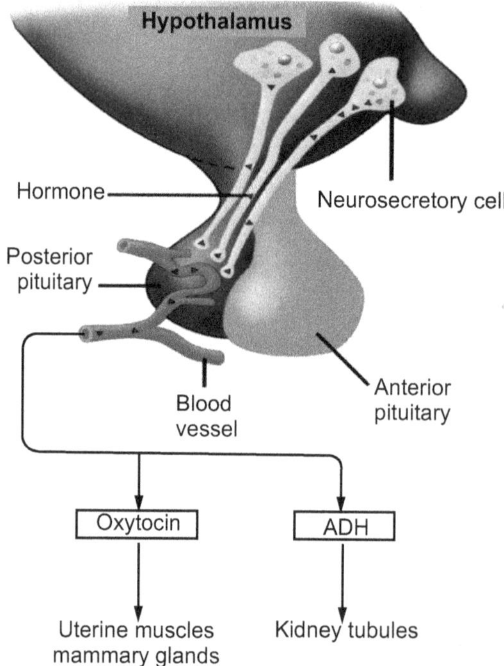

Fig. 6.8: Hormones secreted by posterior pituitary gland

Oxytocin
- During and after childbirth, oxytocin affects two target tissues: the uterus and the breasts.
- During delivery it enhances the contraction of smooth muscle cells in the wall of the uterus
- After childbirth, it stimulates milk ejection from the mammary glands in response to the mechanical stimulus provided by a suckling infant.

Anti-diuretic Hormone (ADH)
- An antidiuretic hormone decreases the urine production.
- ADH causes the kidneys to return more water to the blood, thus decreasing the urine volume.
- ADH also decreases the water lost through sweating and causes the constriction of arterioles, which increases the blood pressure.
- It is also called as vasopressin.
- The amount of ADH secreted varies with blood osmotic pressure and blood volume.

6.6 THYROID GLAND
- It is located in the neck region just below the larynx.
- It weighs approximately 30g.
- It is butterfly shaped, having two lobes joined by isthmus (middle lobe).
- The gland is made up of a large number of follicles called as thyroid follicles.
- The wall of each follicle consists of two types of cells.
    - ✓ Follicular cells
    - ✓ Para-follicular cells
- Follicular cells are present in the lumen of follicles. It is made up of cuboidal epithelial cells.
- The follicular cells secrete thyroxine called as T_4 (4 iodine atoms) and tri-iodo-thyronine or T_3 (3 atoms of iodine).
- T_3 and T_4 are called as thyroid hormones.
- Some cells do not reach the follicle lumen or lie between the follicles. These cells are called as parafollicular cells or C (clear) cells.
- They produce calcitonin that maintains calcium homeostasis.

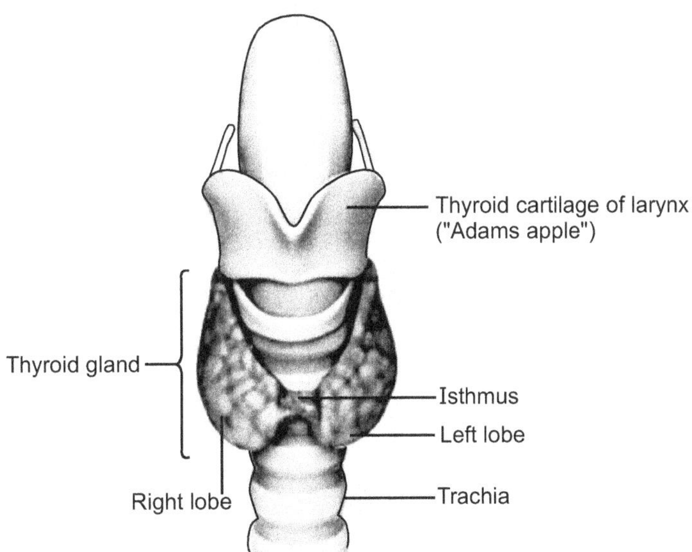

Fig. 6.9: Thyroid gland

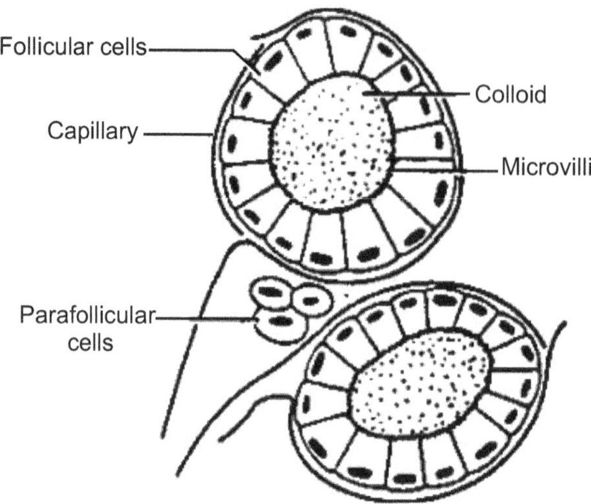

Fig. 6.10: Histology of thyroid follicle

Functions of Thyroid Hormone

Increase in basal metabolic rate

- Thyroid hormone increases the basal metabolic rate.
- 1 gm glucose on oxidation produces 4 calories of energy.
- 1 mg of thyroid hormone on injection releases 1000 calories of energy.

Effect on growth

- T_3 and T_4 promote the physical growth in children, development of skeleton, growth of individual and also promote mental growth.
- It promotes growth and development of brain during foetal life.
- Hypersecretion of thyroid hormone causes mental retardation in children.

Effect on carbohydrate, fat and protein metabolism

- The thyroid hormones stimulate the protein synthesis, increases lipolysis, increase cholesterol excretion in bile and increase the use of glucose for ATP production.

Effect on cardiovascular system

- Thyroid hormones increases the heart rate, cardiac contractility and cardiac output.
- They also promote vasodilation, which leads to enhanced blood flow to many organs.

Effect on central nervous system

- Both decreased and increased concentrations of thyroid hormones lead to alterations in the mental state.
- Low quantity of thyroid hormone causes mental sluggishness in individual, while high quantity causes anxiety and nervousness.

Effects on reproductive system

- Normal reproductive behaviour and physiology depends on normal levels of thyroid hormone.
- Hypothyroidism is associated with infertility condition.

Formation, storage and release of thyroid hormones

- About 50 mg of iodine is required every year to produce normal quantities of thyroid hormone.
- Iodine is stored in the form of thyroglobulin.
- Iodine (in the form of iodides) is absorbed from GIT and it enters the circulation.
- After absorption iodine has two fates:
  - ✓ It is excreted in urine or
  - ✓ It is taken up by the basal membrane of the thyroid cell.

1. **Iodide trapping:** Thyroid follicular cells trap iodide ions (I^-) by actively transporting them from the blood into the cytosol.

2. **Synthesis of thyroglobulin:** Follicular cells after trapping I^- ions, synthesise thyroglobulin (TGB), a large glycoprotein produced in the rough endoplasmic reticulum. It is then modified in the Golgi complex and packaged into secretory vesicles. The vesicles later undergo exocytosis and release TGB into the lumen of the follicle.

3. **Oxidation of iodide:** Some of the amino acids in TGB are tyrosines and these become iodinated. However, negatively charged iodide ions cannot bind to tyrosine until they undergo oxidation to iodine: $2\,I \rightarrow I_2$. As the iodide ions are being oxidised, they pass through the membrane into the lumen of the follicle.

4. **Iodination of tyrosine:** As iodine molecules (I_2) form, they react with tyrosine. Binding of one iodine atom yields mono-iodo-tyrosine (T_1), and a second iodination produces di-iodo-tyrosine (T_2). The TGB with attached iodine atoms accumulate and is stored in the lumen of the thyroid follicle. This is called as colloid.

5. **Coupling of T_1 and T_2:** During the last step in the synthesis of thyroid hormone, two T_2 molecules join to form T_4 or one T_1 and one T_2 join to form T_3.

6. **Pinocytosis and digestion of colloid:** Droplets of colloid re-enter the follicular cells by pinocytosis and merge with lysosomes. Digestive enzymes in the lysosomes break down TGB, cleaving off molecules of T_3 and T_4.

7. **Secretion of thyroid hormones:** Because T_3 and T_4 are lipid soluble, they diffuse through the plasma membrane into interstitial fluid and then into the blood. T_4 normally is secreted in greater quantity than T_3, but T_3 is several times more potent. Moreover, after T_4 enters a body cell, most of it is converted to T_3 by removal of one iodine.

8. **Transport in the blood:** More than 99% of T_3 and the T_4 combine with transport proteins in the blood, mainly thyroxine-binding globulin (TBG).

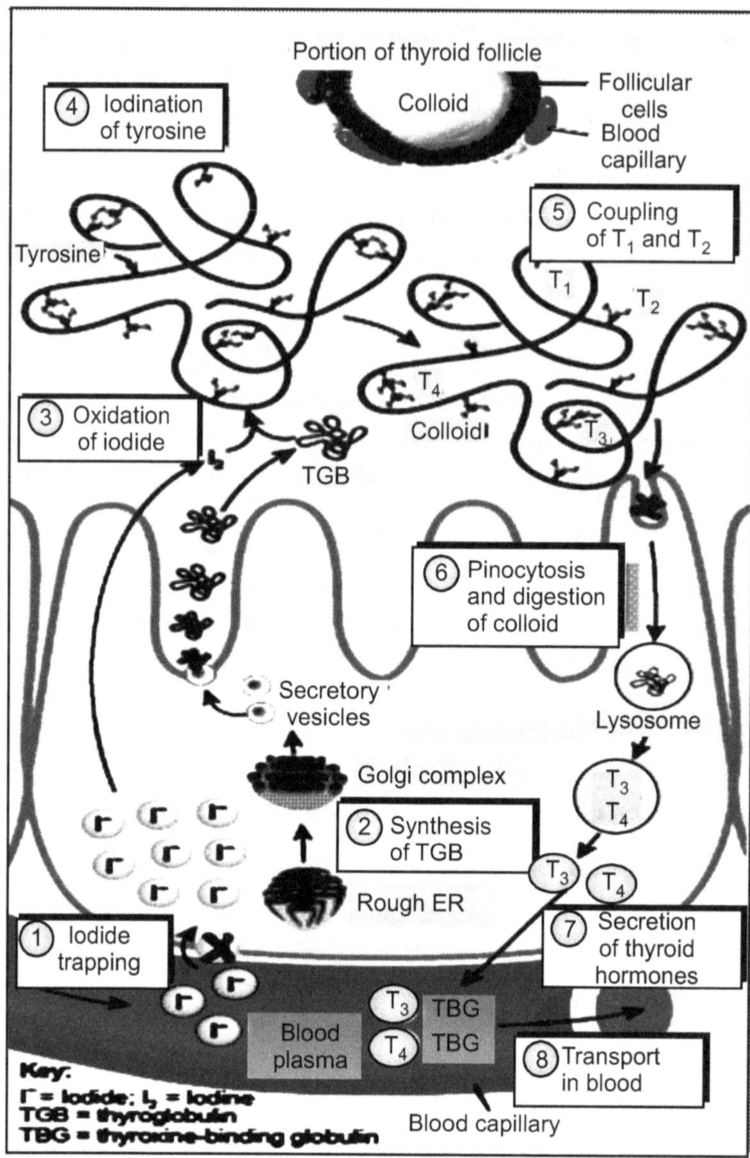

Fig. 6.11: Formation, storage and release of thyroid hormones

Calcitonin

- It is secreted by the parafollicular or C-cells in the thyroid gland.
- It acts on bone and kidneys to reduce the blood calcium (Ca^{2+}) level when it is raised.
- It reduces the reabsorption of calcium ions from the bones and inhibits reabsorption of calcium by the renal tubules.
- Its effect is opposite to that of parathyroid hormone which is secreted by the parathyroid glands.
- Release of calcitonin is stimulated by an increase in the blood calcium level.

- When blood calcium level is high, calcitonin lowers the amount of blood calcium and phosphates by inhibiting bone resorption by osteoclasts and by accelerating the uptake of calcium and phosphates into bone extracellular matrix.

6.7 PARATHYROID GLAND

- There are four small parathyroid glands, two embedded in the posterior surface of each lobe of the thyroid gland.
- It weighs approximately 40 mg.
- Histologically, it contains two kinds of epithelial cells.
- The more abundant cells are the chief cells which produce parathyroid hormone (PTH).
- The other type of cell is oxyphil cell; its function is not known.
- Parathyroid hormone is the major regulator of the levels of calcium (Ca^{2+}), magnesium (Mg^{2+}) and phosphate (HPO_4^{2-}) ions in the blood.
- The result is elevated bone resorption, which releases calcium (Ca^{2+}) and phosphates (HPO_4^{2-}) into the blood.
- Parathormone and calcitonin from the thyroid gland maintain the blood calcium levels within the normal range which is needed for muscle contraction, blood clotting and nerve impulse transmission.

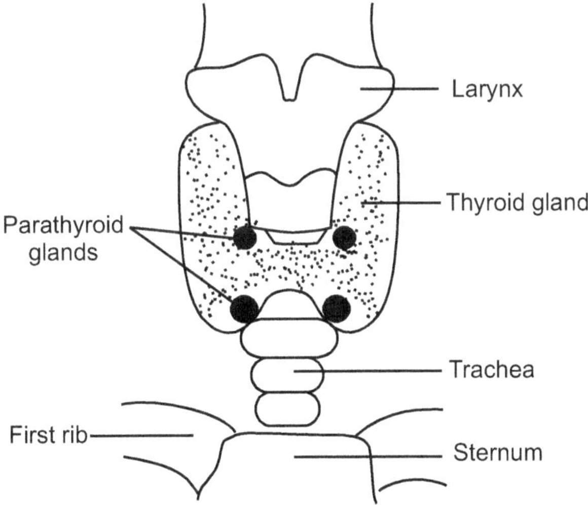

Fig. 6.12: Parathyroid gland

6.8 ADRENAL GLAND

- The paired adrenal (suprarenal) glands lie on top of the kidney.
- Adrenal gland is 3–5 cm in height, 2–3 cm in width and 1 cm thick.
- Its weight is 3.5–5 g.

- It is divided into two parts
  - ✓ **Adrenal cortex:** 80–90% of the gland, peripheral portion
  - ✓ **Adrenal medulla:** 20% of the gland, central portion
- **Adrenal cortex:** It is subdivided into three zones each of which secretes different hormones.
  - ✓ **Zona glomerulosa:** The outer zone just below the connective tissue capsule. Its cells secrete mineralocorticoid hormones.
  - ✓ **Zona fasciculata:** It is the middle zone. Its cells secrete glucocorticoid hormone.
  - ✓ **Zona reticularis:** It is the inner zone. Its cells secrete androgens (steroid hormones).
- **Adrenal medulla:** It is the inner region of the adrenal gland. It is made up of chromaffin cells. The two major hormones synthesised by the adrenal medulla are:
  - ✓ Epinephrine (Adrenaline)
  - ✓ Norepinephrine (Noradrenalin)

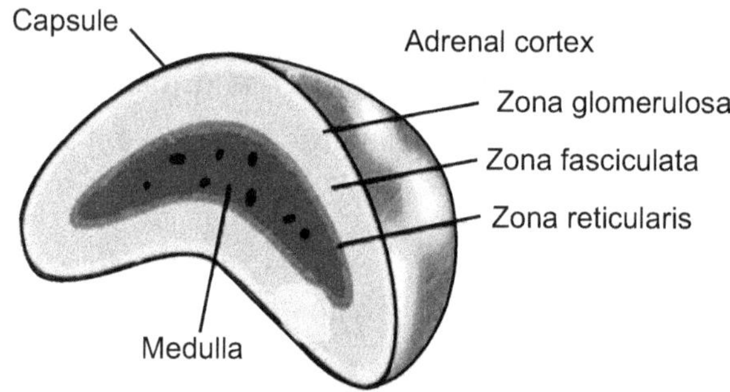

Fig. 6.13: Adrenal gland

Mineralocorticoids

These are a class of steroid hormones characterised by their ability to regulate concentrations of sodium and potassium ions in the extracellular fluids. Mineralocorticoids play a critical role in maintaining the electrolyte and fluid balance of the body. The principal steroid with mineralocorticoid activity is aldosterone.

Aldosterone

- Aldosterone is the major mineralocorticoid.
- It regulates homeostasis of sodium ions and potassium ions and helps in regulating blood pressure and blood volume.
- Aldosterone also promotes the excretion of hydrogen ions in the urine which can help in preventing the acidosis.

Renin-angiotensin-aldosterone (RAA) System

Refer Article 5.9 of Chapter 5.

Glucocorticoids

Glucocorticoids are steroids that have anti inflammatory property. GC's interrupt inflammation by suppressing the proteins that promote inflammation. Glucocorticoids help mediate the stress response and help re-establish the homeostasis. They also help the body respond to environmental change. GCs also affect metabolism by causing cells in the liver to make more sugar.

Different glucocorticoids secreted by adrenal cortex include:

- ✓ Cortisol
- ✓ Corticosterone
- ✓ Cortisone
- ✓ Prednisone
- ✓ Methyl prednisone
- ✓ Dexamethasone

Effects of Glucocorticoids

Protein breakdown

- It increases the rate of protein breakdown in muscle fibres and thus increases the liberation of amino acids into the bloodstream. The amino acids are used for the synthesis of new proteins or for ATP synthesis.

Glucose formation

- Glucocorticoid stimulates the liver cells and converts certain amino acids to glucose which is used for ATP production.

Lipolysis

- Glucocorticoids stimulate lipolysis, the breakdown of triglycerides and release of fatty acids from adipose tissue into the blood vessels.

Anti-inflammatory effects

- Glucocorticoids inhibit white blood cells that participate in inflammatory responses. Glucocorticoids are very useful in the treatment of rheumatoid arthritis.

Depression of immune responses

- High doses of glucocorticoids depress immune responses. For this reason, glucocorticoids are prescribed for organ transplant recipients to retard tissue rejection by the immune system.

Resistance to stress

- Glucocorticoid provides resistance to stress. It is used to combat a range of stress, including exercise, fasting, fright, temperature extremes, high altitude, bleeding, infection, surgery, trauma and disease.

Sex hormones (Androgen)

- It is a steroid hormone that stimulates or controls the development and maintenance of male characteristics by binding to androgen receptors.
- This includes the activity of the accessory male sex organs and development of male secondary sex characteristics.

- In both males and females, the adrenal cortex secretes small amounts of androgens.
- The major androgen secreted by the adrenal gland is dehydroepiandrosterone (DHEA).
- After puberty in males, the androgen testosterone is released in much greater quantity by the testes.
- In females adrenal androgens play an important role.
- They promote libido (sex drive) and are converted into estrogens (feminizing sex steroids) by other body tissues.
- Adrenal androgens also stimulate growth of axillary and pubic hair in boys and girls.

6.9 PANCREAS

- It is both an endocrine gland as well as an exocrine gland.
- It measures about 12.5–15 cm in length.
- The pancreas is located in the curve of the duodenum, the first part of the small intestine.
- It consists of a head, a body and a tail.
- Pancreas is functionally divided into two parts.
  - ✓ **Exocrine pancreas:** The pancreas is made up of small clusters of glandular epithelium cells, about 99% are arranged in clusters called as acini and constitute exocrine portion of the organ. The cells within the acini secrete a mixture of fluid and digestive enzymes called as the pancreatic juice.
  - ✓ **Endocrine pancreas:** Remaining 1% of the cells are arranged into clusters called as pancreatic islets (islets of Langerhans). The cells secrete the hormone insulin, glucagon which is responsible for the maintenance of blood sugar level. Insulin lowers the blood sugar level whereas, glucagon increases the blood sugar level.

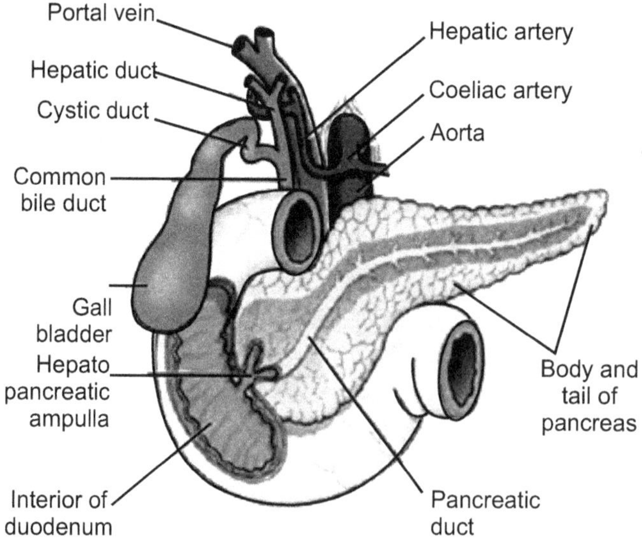

Fig. 6.14: Pancreas and associated structures

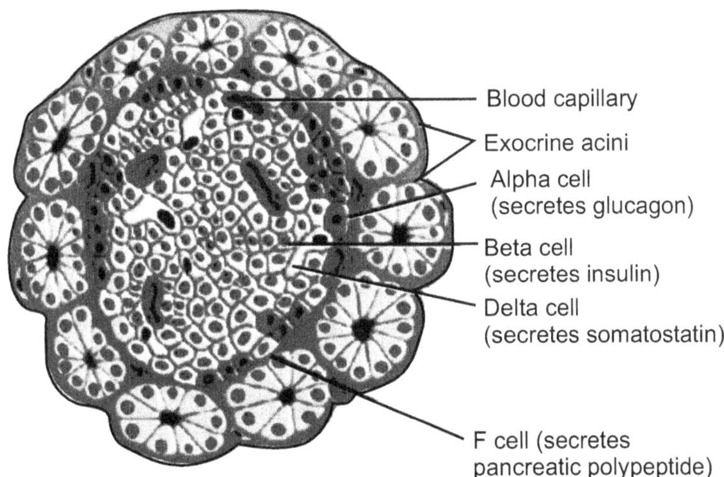

Fig. 6.15: Pancreatic islet and surrounding acini

Cell in Pancreatic Islets

- It contains four types of hormone-secreting cells:
  - ✓ **Alpha or A cells:** It constitutes about 17% of pancreatic islet cells and secretes glucagon.
  - ✓ **Beta or B cells:** It constitutes about 70% of pancreatic islet cells and secretes insulin.
  - ✓ **Delta or D cells:** It constitutes about 7% of pancreatic islet cells and secretes somatostatin.
  - ✓ **F cells:** It constitutes the remainder of pancreatic islet cells and secretes pancreatic polypeptide.

Glucagon

- It is secreted from alpha cells of the pancreatic islets.
- **Secretion:** Decreased blood level of glucose, exercise and mainly protein meals stimulate the secretion of glucagon. Somatostatin and insulin inhibit the glucagon secretion.
- **Action:** It raises the blood glucose levels by accelerating breakdown of glucagon into glucose in liver (glycogenolysis), converting other nutrients into glucose in the liver (gluconeogenesis) and releasing glucose into the blood.

Insulin

- It is secreted from the beta cells of pancreatic islets.
- **Secretion:** Increased blood level of glucose, glucagon, human growth hormone (HGH) and adrenocorticotropin hormone (ACTH) stimulates secretion.
- **Action:** It lowers elevated blood glucose level by accelerating transport of glucose into cells converting glucose into glycogen (glycogenesis) and decreasing glycogenolysis and gluconeogenesis.

Somatostatin

- It is secreted by the delta cells of pancreatic islets.

- **Secretion:** Pancreatic polypeptide inhibits secretion.
- **Action:** It inhibits secretion of insulin and glucagon and slows absorption of nutrients from the GIT.

Pancreatic polypeptide

- It is secreted from F cells of pancreatic islets.
- **Secretion:** Meals containing protein, fasting, exercise and acute hypoglycaemia stimulate secretion. Somatostatin and elevated blood glucose level inhibit secretion.
- **Action:** It inhibits secretion of somatostatin and gall bladder contraction. It promotes the secretion of pancreatic digestive enzymes.

6.10 PINEAL GLAND

- It is a small endocrine gland attached to the roof of third ventricle of the brain.
- It is about 10 mm long, reddish brown in colour and is surrounded by a capsule.
- The gland consists of masses of neuroglia and secretory cells called as pinealocytes.
- The pineal gland secretes melatonin, an amine hormone derived from serotonin.
- Melatonin is useful in:
  - ✓ Coordination of the circadian rhythms.
  - ✓ Inhibition of growth and development of the sex organs before puberty, possibly by preventing synthesis or release of gonadotropins.

6.11 GONADS (TESTES AND OVARIES)

- Gonads are the organs that produce gametes-sperm in males and oocytes in females.
- The ovaries are paired oval bodies located in the female pelvic cavity, produce steroid hormones including estrogens (estradiol and estrone) and progesterone.
- These female sex hormones, along with FSH and LH from the anterior pituitary, regulate the menstrual cycle, maintain pregnancy and prepare the mammary glands for lactation.
- They also promote enlargement of the breasts and widening of the hips at puberty, and help maintain these female secondary sex characteristics.
- The ovaries also produce inhibin, a protein hormone that inhibits the secretion of follicle-stimulating hormone (FSH).
- During pregnancy, the ovaries and placenta produce a peptide hormone called as relaxin, that increases the flexibility of the pubic symphysis during pregnancy and helps dilate the uterine cervix during labour and delivery.
- The male gonads called the testes are oval glands that lie in the scrotum.
- The main hormone produced and secreted by the testes is testosterone or male sex hormone.
- Testosterone stimulates the production of sperm and stimulates the development and maintenance of male secondary sex characteristics, such as growth of beard and deepening of the voice.
- The testes also produce inhibin, which inhibits secretion of FSH.

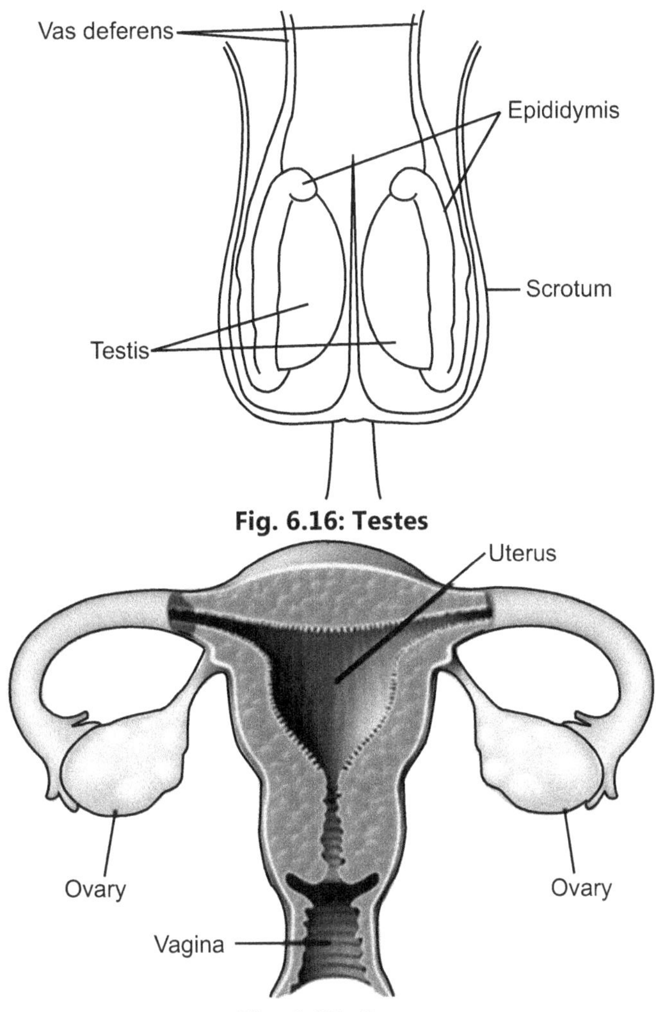

Fig. 6.16: Testes

Fig. 6.17: Ovary

6.12 DISORDERS OF THE ENDOCRINE SYSTEM

I.   Pituitary Gland Disorders

Pituitary dwarfism

- Hyposecretion of human growth hormone during the growing years of an individual, slows bone growth and overall rate of growth. This condition is called as pituitary dwarfism.

- In pituitary dwarfism, height is stunted, but slow is growth of rest of the body, resulting in a perfectly proportioned short individual. Hence, pituitary dwarfism is sometimes called as proportionate dwarfism.

- Treatment requires the administration of human growth hormone during the childhood.

Pituitary gigantism

- Hypersecretions of human growth hormone during childhood before the fusion of the epiphyseal growth plates leads to gigantism.

- It may occur at any age and has been observed as early as the first six to nine months of age.
- It results in an abnormal increase in the length of long bones.
- The person grows to be very tall but the body proportions are about normal.

Pituitary acromegaly

- Hypersecretions of human growth hormone during adulthood causes acromegaly i.e. after complete epiphyseal fusion
- At this age as the epiphyses of the long bones are fused with the shaft the person cannot grow taller, but the soft tissues continue to grow and bones grow in thickness.
- Acromegalic patients are at increased risk of developing other tumours or lesions of the body.

Diabetes insipidus

- The most common abnormality associated with dysfunction of the posterior pituitary is diabetes insipidus.
- This disorder is due to defects in antidiuretic hormone (ADH) receptors or an inability to secrete ADH.
- Two types of diabetes insipidus are:
  - ✓ **Neurogenic diabetes insipidus:** It results from hyposecretion of ADH, usually caused by a brain tumour, head trauma or brain surgery that damages the posterior pituitary or the hypothalamus.
  - ✓ **Nephrogenic diabetes insipidus:** The kidneys do not respond to ADH. The ADH receptors may be non-functional or the kidneys may be damaged.
- The common symptoms are excretion of large volumes of urine, results in dehydration and thirst.

II. Thyroid Disorders

Cretinism

- Extreme hyposecretion of thyroid hormone during foetal life, infancy or childhood leads to cretinism.
- In absence of thyroid hormones, the skeleton fails to grow and mature
- This condition results in severely stunted physical and mental growth
- The skin is thick, flabby and waxy in colour, the nose is flattened, the abdomen protrudes and there is a general slowness of movement and speech.

Myxedema

- Hypothyroidism during the adulthood produces myxedema which occurs about five times more often in females than in males.
- The characteristic of this disorder is edema (accumulation of interstitial fluid) that causes the facial tissues to swell and look puffy.

Grave's disease

- The most common form of hyperthyroidism is Graves disease which also occurs 7 to 10 times more often in females than in males, usually before the age of 40.
- In this disease, the thyroid gland increases two or three times the normal size and produces more amount of thyroid hormone.
- The patients often have a peculiar edema behind the eyes called as exophthamos which causes the eyes to protrude.

Goiter

- It is simply an enlargement of the thyroid gland.
- It may be associated with hyperthyroidism, hypothyroidism or euthyroidism which means normal secretion of thyroid hormone.
- In some places in the world, dietary iodine intake is inadequate.
- The resultant low level of thyroid hormone in the blood stimulates secretion of TSH which causes the thyroid gland enlargement.

III. Adrenal Gland Disorders

Cushing syndrome

- Hypersecretions of cortisol by the adrenal cortex produces Cushing syndrome.
- The causes include a tumour of the adrenal gland that secrete cortisol or a tumour that secrete adrenocorticotropic hormone which in turn stimulates excessive secretion of cortisol.
- The characteristic feature of this syndrome is a fatty hump between shoulders, a rounded face and pink or purple stretch marks on skin.
- Cushing syndrome can also result in high blood pressure, bone loss and diabetes.

Addison's disease

- Hyposecretion of glucocorticoids and aldosterone causes Addison's disease (chronic adrenocortical insufficiency).
- Low aldosterone level leads to elevated potassium and decreased sodium level in the blood, low blood pressure, dehydration, decreased cardio output and even cardiac arrest.

Pheochromocytomas

- Benign tumours of the chromaffin cells of the adrenal medulla called as Pheochromocytomas cause hypersecretion of epinephrine and norepinephrine.
- The symptoms are rapid heart rate, high blood pressure, high levels of glucose in blood and urine, an elevated basal metabolic rate (BMR), flushed face, nervousness, sweating and decreased gastrointestinal motility.

IV. Pancreatic Islet Disorders

Diabetes mellitus

- It is a group of metabolic diseases in which a person has high blood sugar, either because the pancreas does not produce enough insulin or cells do not respond to the insulin.
- The most common endocrine disorder is diabetes mellitus, caused by an inability to produce or use insulin from the beta cells of Langerhans.
- It can be characterised by:
  - ✓ Hyperglycaemia: Increased blood glucose level
  - ✓ Glucosuria: Loss of glucose in urine
  - ✓ Polyuria: Excessive thirst
  - ✓ Polyphagia: Excessive eating
- Diabetes mellitus is of two types
  - ✓ Type-I (IDDM): It is also called as insulin-dependent diabetes. It is an autoimmune condition that often begins in the childhood. It's caused by the body's antibodies attacking its own pancreas. The damaged pancreas does not make insulin.
  - ✓ Type-II (NIDDM): It is also called as non-insulin-dependent or adult-onset diabetes. In this case, the pancreas usually produces insulin, but either the amount produced is not enough for the body's needs or the body's cells are resistant to it.

QUESTIONS

Short Answer Questions:

1. Give the difference between circulating hormone and local hormone.
2. Write a note on hormone released from pineal gland.
3. Write a note on hormones of pituitary glands and its function.
4. Give location, hormones secreted by and functions of pituitary gland, thyroid gland and adrenal gland.
5. Write a note on hypothalamic hormone.
6. Explain synthesis, storage and release of thyroid hormone.
7. Write a note on mechanism of hormone.
8. Explain the role of hormones of pituitary gland.
9. Explain the physiological role of hormones of anterior pituitary gland.
10. Enlist various hormones secreted by various endocrine glands with their functions.
11. Explain the physiological role of FSH and LH.
12. Explain the hormones released from thyroid gland.
13. Write a note on Renin-Angiotensin-Aldosterone System.

Long Answer Questions:

1. Explain the mechanism of water soluble and lipid soluble hormone action.
2. Write a note on hormone released from hypothalamus and pituitary gland.
3. Explain the process of formation, storage and release of thyroid hormones.

UNIT V

Chapter 7 ...

REPRODUCTIVE SYSTEM

◆ LEARNING OBJECTIVES ◆

❖ To describe the structure and functions of organs of the male reproductive system.

❖ To discuss the process of spermatogenesis in the testes.

❖ To describe the structure, and functions of organs of the female reproductive system.

❖ To discuss the process of oogenesis in the ovaries.

❖ To explain the female reproductive cycle.

7.1 INTRODUCTION

The reproductive system is a system of sex organs which work together for the purpose of sexual reproduction. The male and female reproductive organs although completely different in structure and function work together to produce offspring.

Gynecology is the branch of medicine concerned with the diagnosis and treatment of diseases of the female reproductive system.

Andrology is the branch of medicine that deals with male disorders, especially infertility and sexual dysfunction.

The production of new living organisms by combining genetic information from two individuals of different sexes is called as sexual reproduction. The union of the male gamete (sperm) with the female gamete (secondary oocytes) results in fertilization. The resulting cell contains one set of chromosomes from each parent. The gonads - testes in males and ovaries in females produce gametes and secrete sex hormones.

7.2 MALE REPRODUCTIVE SYSTEM

The organs of the male reproductive system include;

- The testes-produces sperms and secretes hormones
- A system of ducts (epididymis, ductus deferens, ejaculatory ducts, urethra)
- Accessory sex glands (seminal vesicles, prostate and bulbourethral glands)
- Supporting structures (the scrotum and the penis)

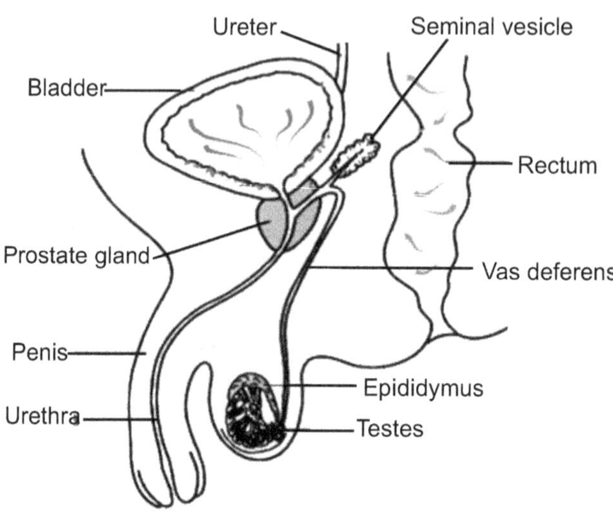

Fig. 7.1: Male reproductive system

7.2.1 Penis

- The penis contains the urethra and is a passageway for the ejaculation of semen and the excretion of urine.
- It is cylindrical in shape and consists of three parts.
    - ✓ Root of penis
    - ✓ Body of penis
    - ✓ Glans penis
- The body of penis is composed of three cylindrical masses of tissue, which is surrounded by fibrous tissue called as tunica albuginea.
- Two dorsoventral masses are called as corpora canvernosa penis.
- The smaller midventeral mass is called as corpus spongiosum penis, which contains spongy urethra and keeps it open during ejaculation.
- The distal end of penis is slightly enlarged and is called as glans penis.
- The glans penis is covered with prepuce or foreskin.
- The urethra opens at glans penis in the form of a slit called as external urethral orifice.
- The root of penis is made up of;
    - ✓ **Bulb of the penis:** The expanded portion of the base of the corpus spongiosum penis
    - ✓ **Crus of the penis:** The two separated and tapered portions of corpora cavernosa penis.
- The penis functions as reproductive organ as well as excretory organ.
- During intercourse, the penis delivers semen into the vagina.
- As an excretory organ, the penis delivers urine out of the body.

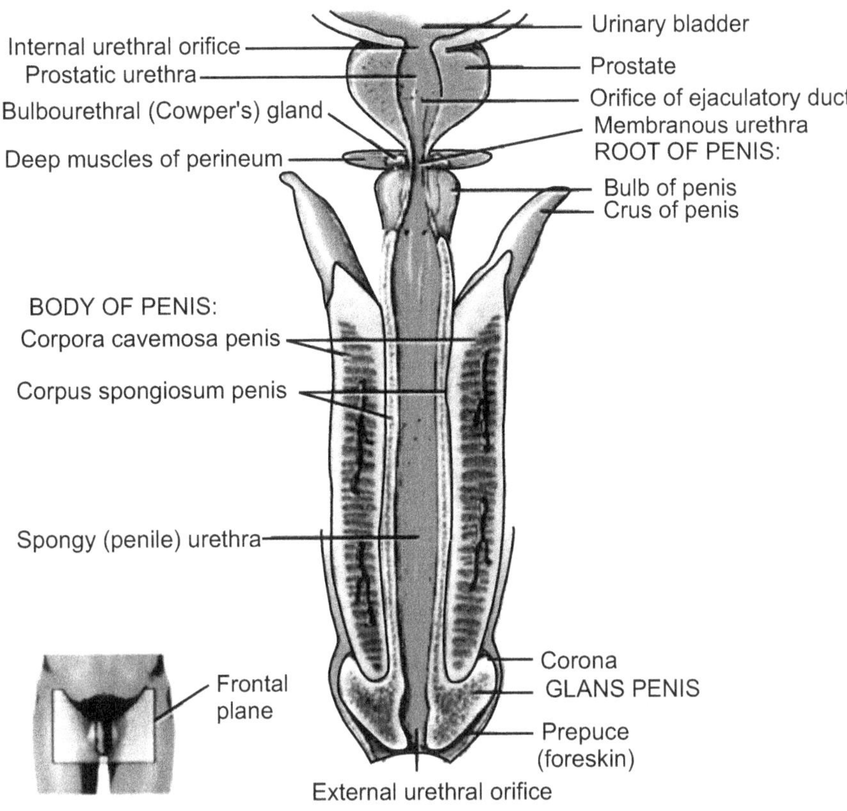

Fig. 7.2: Frontal section of Penis

7.2.2 Scrotum

- It is the supporting structure for testes and consists of loose skin that hangs from the root of the penis.
- Externally the scrotum looks like a single pouch of skin, thin, wrinkled and pigmented.
- Internally the scrotal septum divides the scrotum into two sacs, each containing a single testis.
- Normal sperm production requires a temperature of about 2-3°C below the body temperature.

7.2.3 Testes

- These are paired oval glands in the scrotum about 5 cm in length and 2.5 cm in diameter.
- It weighs approximately 10-15 gm.
- These are suspended in the scrotum by the spermatic cords.
- They are surrounded by three layers of tissue.
  - ✓ Tunica vaginalis
  - ✓ Tunica albuginea
  - ✓ Tunica vasculosa

- **Tunica vaginalis:** This is a double membrane forming the outer covering of testes and derived from the peritoneum.
- **Tunica albuginea:** Internal to the tunica vaginalis is the tunica albuginea composed of dense irregular connective tissue.
- It extends inwards forming septa that divides the testis into a series of internal compartments called as lobules.
- **Tunica vasculosa:** This consists of a network of capillaries supported by delicate connective tissue.
- Each testis consist of 200-300 lobules and within each lobules are 1- 4 convoluted loops composed of germinal epithelial cells called as seminiferous tubules, where sperm are produced.
- The process by which the seminiferous tubules of the testes produce sperm is called as spermatogenesis.
- The seminiferous tubules contain two types of cells.
    - ✓ **Spermatogenic cells:** It is the sperm forming cells.
    - ✓ **Sertoli cells:** It supports spermatogenesis process.
- In the spaces between adjacent seminiferous tubules are clusters of cells called as Leydig cells.
- These cells secrete testosterone, the most common androgen.
- At the upper pole of testes, the tubules combine to form a single tubule.
- This tubule is 6 m in length. It is repeatedly folded and tightly packed into a mass called as epididymis.
- It leaves the scrotum as vas deferens in the spermatic cord.
- Blood and lymph vessels pass to the testes in the spermatic cords.

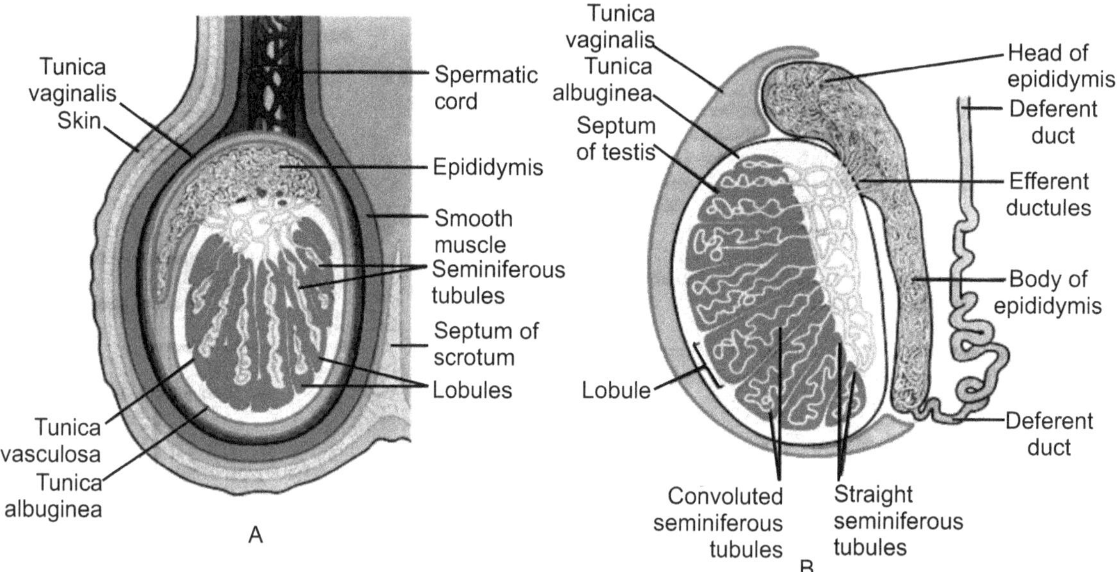

Fig. 7.3: The testis: (A) Section of the testis and its coverings. (B) Longitudinal section of a testis and deferent duct

7.2.4 Sperm

- The process of production of sperms from the testis is called as spermatogenesis.
- Spermatogenesis process produces about 300 million sperms per day.
- Once ejaculated they do not survive for more than 48 hours within female reproductive tract.
- It consist of three parts;
  - ✓ Head
  - ✓ Mid piece (Body)
  - ✓ Tail
- **Head:** It is 4-5 µm long. It contains an acrosome; a lysosome like vesicle and nucleus. It also contains the enzymes required to penetrate the outer layers of the ovum to reach and fuse with its nucleus.
- **Body:** It consists of many mitochondria, which provide ATP for motility into female reproductive system.
- **Tail:** A typical flagellum uses the tail for motility into female reproductive tract. From head to tip of tail, human sperm is about 70 µm in length.

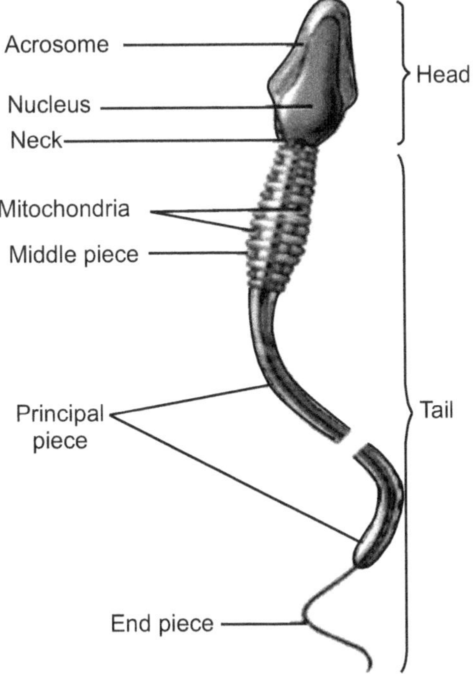

Fig. 7.4: Sperm

7.2.5 Ducts of Testis

- These are the epididymis, ducts (vas) deferens, spermatic cords, ejaculatory ducts and the urethra.

Epididymis

- It is a comma shaped organ of about 4 cm long.
- It consists of 3 parts
  - ✓ **Head:** It is the larger, superior portion of epididymis.
  - ✓ **Body:** It is the narrow mid-portion of the epididymis.
  - ✓ **Tail:** It is the smaller and inferior portion.
- Each epididymis consists of tightly coiled of the epididymis.
- It is the site for sperm maturation- the process by which sperm acquires motility and the ability to fertilise the ovum.
- It also helps to propel sperm into the vas deferens during sexual arousal.
- It also stores sperm, which remain viable for up to several months.

Ductus (vas) Deferens

- It starts from epididymis which is about 45 cm long.
- The vas deferens conveys sperm during sexual arousal from the epididymis towards the urethra by peristaltic contraction of muscular coat.
- It also stores sperms for several months.

Spermatic Cords

- The spermatic cords suspend the testes in the scrotum.
- Each cord contains testicular artery, testicular veins, lymphatic vessels, a deferent duct, and testicular nerves to form the cord.

Ejaculatory Ducts

- These are located posterior to the urinary bladder.
- They are 2 cm long..
- They eject sperm into the urethra before ejaculation.

Urethra

- It is a common passageway for urine and semen.
- It is 20 cm long.
- It passes through the prostrate, urogenital diaphragm and the penis.
- It is divided into 3 parts
  - ✓ **Prostatic Urethra:** It is 2-3 cm long and passes through the prostrate.
  - ✓ **Membranes Urethra:** Is the shortest, narrowest part and extends from prostrate gland to the bulbs of penis.
  - ✓ **Spongy (Penile) urethra:** It is 15-20 cm long. It ends at external urethral orifice.

7.2.6 Accessory Sex Glands

- The ducts of the male reproductive system store and transport sperm cells, but the accessory gland secretes most of the liquid portion of semen.

- The primary function of the accessory sex glands is to produce seminal fluid to cleanse and lubricate the urethra.
- It includes:
  - ✓ Seminal vesicles
  - ✓ Prostrate
  - ✓ Bulbourethral glands

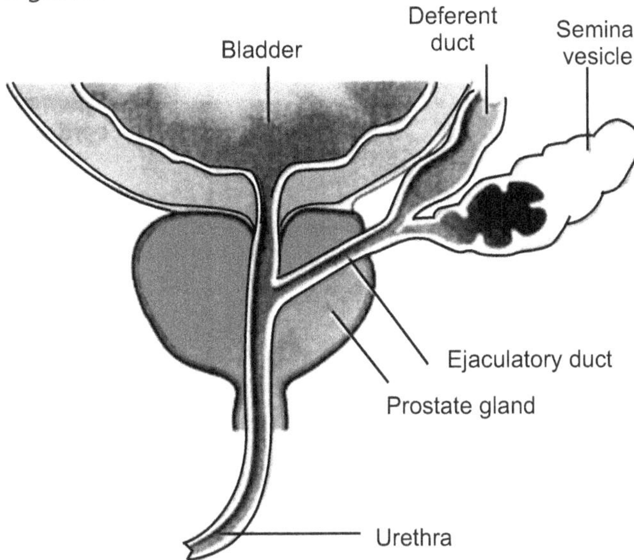

Fig. 7.5: Accessory sex glands

Seminal vesicle

- These are paired elongated saclike glands.
- They secrete fluid contents into the ejaculatory ducts of the male reproductive system.
- It secretes a thick, milky, slightly acidic fluid (pH 6.5) that constitutes the bulk of the seminal fluid (semen).
- It contains fructose, proteins, citric acid, inorganic phosphorus, potassium and prostaglandins.
- **Citric acid:** It is used for ATP production by the sperm.
- **Proteolytic enzymes (pepsinogen, lysosomes, amylase and hyaluronidase):** It breaks down the clotting proteins in the seminal vesicles.
- **Acid phosphates:** Its function is unknown.
- **Seminal plasmin:** It is an antibiotic that destroys bacteria.
- **Fructose:** It acts as main energy source for the sperm outside the body.
- **Prostaglandins:** It aids fertilisation by causing the mucous lining of the cervix to be more receptive to sperm. It aides the movement of the sperm towards the ovum due to peristaltic contractions of the uterus and fallopian tubes.
- Prostatic fluid provides a nutritive medium for gametes.

Prostrate Gland

- It is a walnut-sized gland.
- It is located between the bladder and the penis.
- The prostrate lies just in front of the rectum.
- The prostrate continues to grow throughout the life, but grows very slowly after the age of twenty-five.
- The urethra runs through the center of the prostrate, from the bladder to the penis, allowing urine to flow out of the body.
- The prostrate secretes fluid that nourishes and protects sperm.
- During ejaculation, the prostrate squeezes this fluid into the urethra, which is expelled with sperm as semen.
- Men over forty-five may experience an enlargement of the prostrate.

Bulbourethral Gland (Cowper's Gland)

- These are pea sized pair of exocrine glands.
- They are located inferior to the prostrate gland and lateral to the urethra in the urogenital diaphragm.
- They play an important role in the protection of sperm during ejaculation.
- Each Cowper's gland is made of several connected glandular lobules.
- Many tiny hollow tubules spread through each.
- A thin fibrous membrane surrounds the lobules and holds the gland together to give a firm structure to the gland.
- The many lobules meet at an 2.5 cm long duct that carries the secretions of the gland to the urethra.
- In response to sexual stimulation, the Cowper's glands produce an alkaline mucous secretion known as pre-ejaculate.
- The pre-ejaculate neutralises the acidic urine that may still be present in the urethra
- It also lubricates the urethra and external urethral orifice to protect the sperm from mechanical damage during ejaculation.

7.2.7 Semen

- It is a mixture of sperm and seminal fluid that consists of the secretion of seminiferous tubule, seminal vesicle, prostrate and bulbourethral glands.
- The volume of semen in typical ejaculation is 2.5-5 ml with 50-150 million sperms/ml.
- When the number falls below 20 million/ml the male is likely to be infertile.
- A large number is required for successful fertilisation because only a tiny fraction reaches the secondary oocytes.
- The pH of semen is slightly alkaline 7.2-7.7.
- The prostatic secretion gives semen milky appearance, whereas fluid from the seminal vesicles and bulbourethral glands give it a sticky consistency.

- Semen also contains seminal plasmin, an antibiotic that can destroy certain bacteria.
- Seminal plasmin helps to decrease the bacteria in the semen and in the lower female reproductive tract.
- Once ejaculated, it coagulates within 5 min due to presence of clotting proteins from the seminal vesicles.

7.2.8 Spermatogenesis

- In humans spermatogenesis process takes about 65 to 75 days.
- The seminiferous tubule contains large number of germinal epithelial cells called as spermatagonia.
- Spermatogonia contain diploid (2n) number of chromosome.
- Spermatogonia are stem cells.
- After mitosis, one daughter cell remains near the basement membrane of the seminiferous tubule in an undifferentiated state.
- Other daughter cell loses contact with the basement membrane and differentiates into primary spermatocyte.
- Primary spermatocytes are diploid (2n), they have 40 chromosomes.
- Each primary spermatocyte enlarges and undergoes meiosis.
- In meiosis-I, DNA replicates to form two haploid secondary spermatocytes.
- The two cells formed by meiosis-I are called as secondary spermatocytes.
- Each spermatocyte has 23 chromosomes, the haploid number. (Each chromosome within secondary spermatocytes is made up of two chromatids i.e two copies of DNA).
- In meiosis-II no further replication of DNA occurs.
- The secondary spermatocytes undergo further nuclear division (equatorial division) to form 4 haploid cells called as spermatids.
- Therefore, primary spermatocytes produce 4 spermatids via two rounds of cell division (meiosis-I and II).
- Spermiogenesis is the maturation of haploid spermatids into sperm.
- Because, no cell division occurs in spermiogenesis, each spermatid develops into a single sperm cell.
- During this process, spherical spermatids transforms into elongated, slender sperm.
- An acrosome forms a cap like structure of the nucleus, a flagellum develops and mitochondria multiply.
- Finally sperms are released from their connection to sertoli cells. This is called as spermiation.

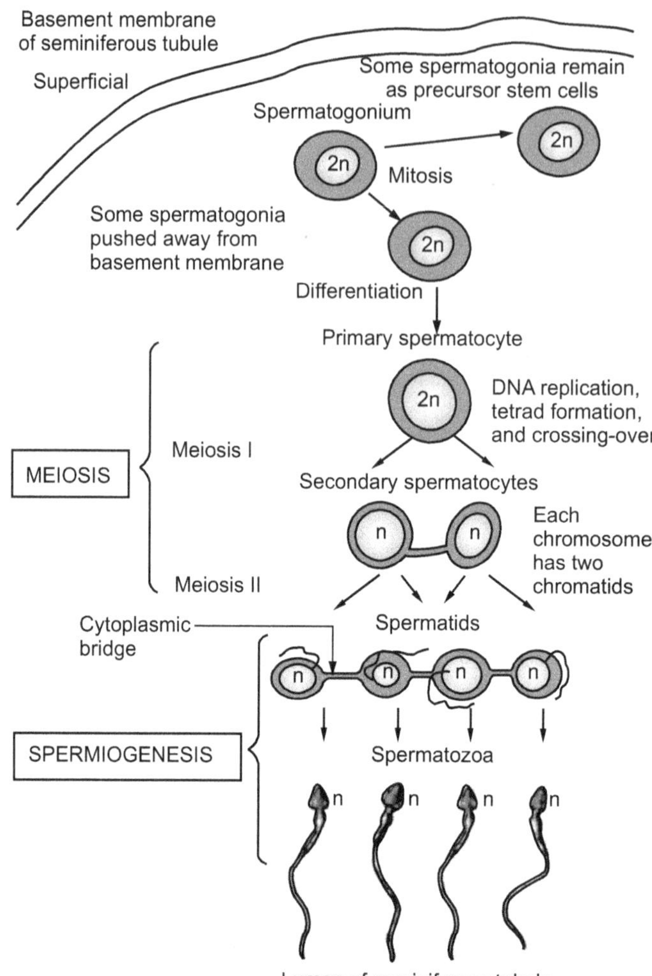

Fig. 7.6: Process of Spermatogenesis

7.3 HORMONES SECRETED BY TESTES

- At puberty certain hypothalamic neurosecretory cells increases the secretion of gonadotropin-releasing hormone (GnRH).
- This hormone stimulates gonadotrophs in the anterior pituitary.
- They are responsible for the secretion of two hormones.
  - ✓ Luteinizing hormone (LH)
  - ✓ Follicle stimulating hormone (FSH)
- LH stimulates Leydig cells located between the seminiferous tubules to secrete the hormone testosterone.
- In some target cells, such as prostrate and seminal vesicles the enzyme 5 α-reductase converts testosterone to another androgen called as dihydrotestosterone (DHT).
- FSH acts indirectly to stimulate spermatogenesis.
- FSH and testosterone act synergistically on the sertoli cells to stimulate secretion of androgen - binding protein (ABP) into the lumen of seminiferous tubules and into the interstitial fluid around the spermatogenic cells. ABP binds to testosterone and keeps the concentration of testosterone high near the seminiferous tubules.
- Testosterone stimulates the spermatogenesis process.

- Once the degree of spermatogenesis required for male reproductive functions have been achieved, sertoli cells release inhibin.
- Inhibin inhibits the secretion of the hormones needed for spermatogenesis.
- Testosterone is necessary for proper physical development in boys.
- Secondary sex characteristics are features that appear during puberty.
- Testosterone is responsible for the development of the following features;
  - ✓ Male pattern development (Before birth)
  - ✓ Enlargement of male sex organs and expression of male secondary sex characteristics (starting of puberty)
  - ✓ Growth of the Adam's apple
  - ✓ Increase in muscle mass
  - ✓ Increase in height
  - ✓ Growth of facial and body hair
  - ✓ Maintaining libido
  - ✓ Sperm production
  - ✓ Maintaining muscle strength and mass
  - ✓ Promoting healthy bone density

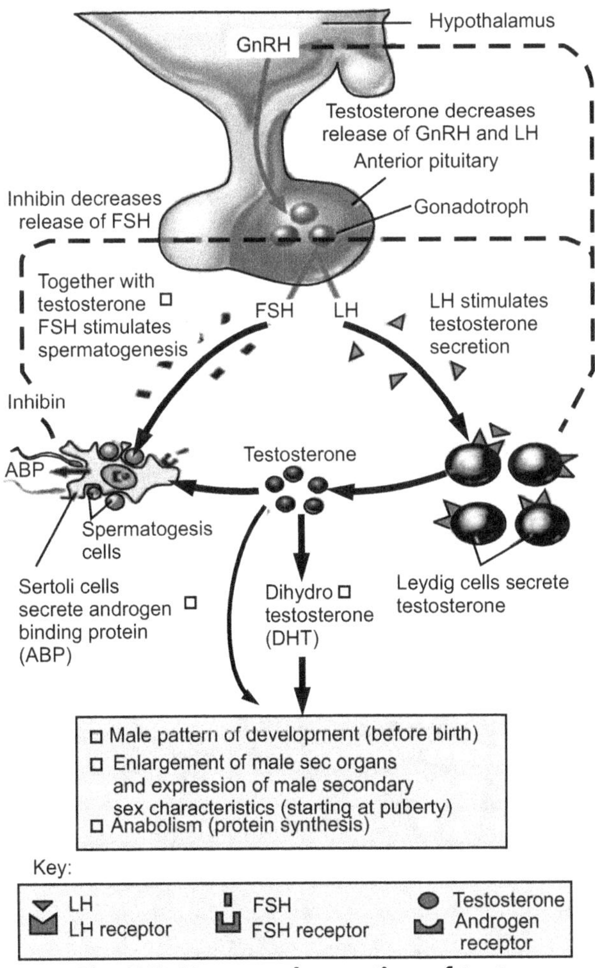

Fig. 7.7: Hormonal secretion of testes

7.4 FEMALE REPRODUCTIVE SYSTEM

It performs the following function:

✓ The ovaries produce secondary oocytes and hormones including progesterone, estrogen, inhibin and relaxin.

✓ Uterine tubes transport secondary oocytes to the uterus and act as site for fertilization.

✓ Reception of spermatozoa.

✓ Provision of suitable environment for fertilisation and foetal development.

✓ Parturition (childbirth)

✓ Mammary gland synthesise, secrete and eject milk for nourishment of the newborn

The female reproductive system consists of;

   ✓ Ovaries (Female gonads)

   ✓ Uterine tube (Fallopian tubes or oviducts)

   ✓ Uterus

   ✓ Vagina

   ✓ External organs (vulva / pudendum)

   ✓ Mammary glands

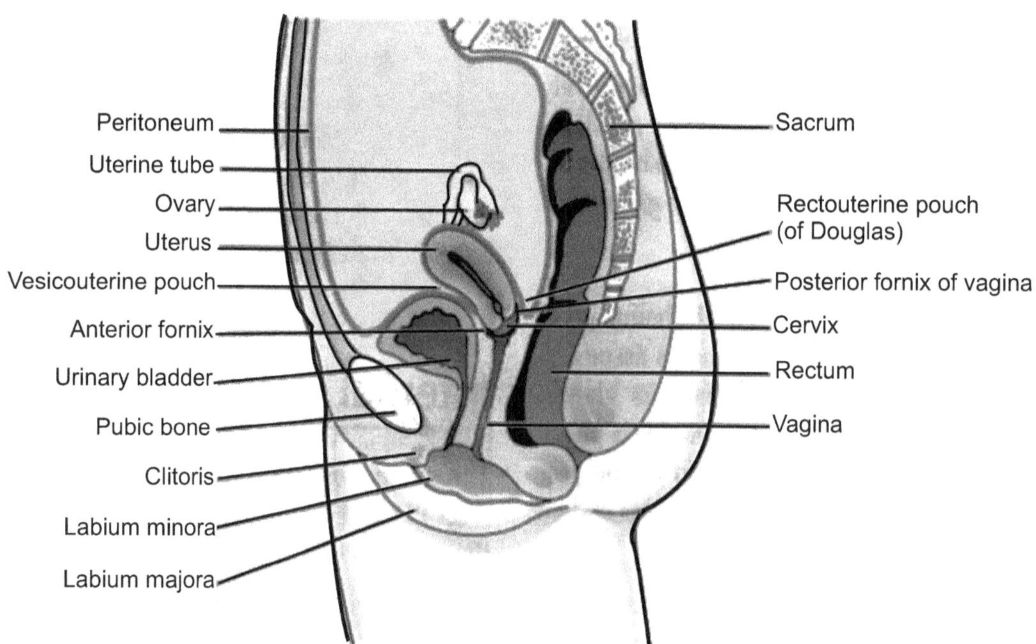

Fig. 7.8: Female reproductive system

7.4.1 Ovaries

- The female gonads are paired glands.
- The ovaries produce:
  - ✓ **Gametes:** It produces secondary oocytes that develop into mature ova (eggs) after fertilisation.
  - ✓ **Hormones:** It secretes various hormones such as progesterone, estrogen, inhibin and relaxin.
- Each ovary lies on each side of uterus.
- They are 2.5 to 3.5 cm long, 2 cm wide and 1 cm thick.
- A series of ligament hold the ovary in position.
  - ✓ **Broad Ligament:** It attaches to the ovaries by a double layered fold of peritoneum called as mesovarian.
  - ✓ **Ovarian Ligament:** It attaches the ovaries to the uterus.
  - ✓ **Suspensory Ligament:** It attaches them to the pelvic cavity.
- Each ovary contains a hilum the point of entrance and exit for blood vessels and nerve.

Histology of Ovary

Each ovary consists of following parts:

- **Germinal epithelium:** It is a large layer of simple epithelium that covers the surface of ovary.
- **Tunica albuginea:** It is a whitish capsule of dense irregular connective tissue located immediately next to the germinal epithelium.
- **Ovarian cortex:** It is present just below the tunica albuginea. It consists of ovarian follicles surrounded by dense irregular connective tissue that contains scattered smooth muscle cells.
- **Ovarian medulla:** It is present deep to the ovarian cortex. Medulla consists of more loosely arranged connective tissue and contains blood vessels, lymphatic vessels and nerves.
- **Ovarian follicles:** It is present in the cortex and consists of oocytes in various stages of development. The surrounding cells nourish the developing oocytes and secrete estrogen as the follicle grows larger.
- **Mature (graafian) follicle:** It is a large, fluid-filled follicle that ruptures to expel the secondary oocytes
- **Corpus Luteum:** It contains the remnants of a mature follicle after ovulation. The corpus luteum produces progesterone, estrogen, relaxin and inhibin until it degenerates into fibrous scar tissue called as corpus albicans.

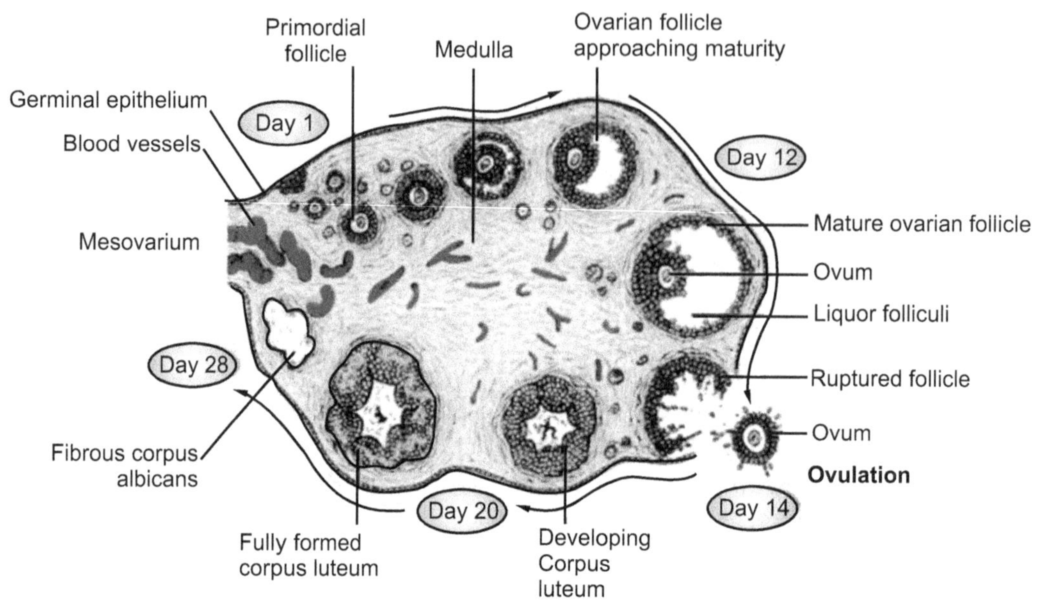

Fig. 7.9: Histology of ovary

7.4.2 Oogenesis

- The formation of gametes in the ovaries is called as oogenesis.
- The cortex of two ovaries contain around 3, 00,000 to 5, 00,000 primary follicles.
- Each primary follicle consists of primary oocyte (ova) which is surrounded by several layers of granulosa cells.
- The primary oocyte is about 100 mm in diameter.
- As primary follicle grows, it forms a clear glycoprotein layer called as zona pellucida between the primary oocyte and the granulosa cells.
- The outermost layers of granulosa cells rest on a basement membrane.
- Encircling the basement membrane is a region called as theca folliculi.
- As primary follicle develops into secondary follicle the theca differentiates into two layers of cells.
  - ✓ Theca interna
  - ✓ Theca externa
- The granulosa cells begin to secrete follicular fluid which builds up in a cavity called as antrum the centre of secondary follicles.
- Innermost layer of granulosa cells becomes firmly attached to the zona pellucida called as corona radiate.
- The secondary follicle becomes larger, turning into a mature graafian follicle.
- The germ cells differentiate into the ovaries to form oogonia (2n) which divide to form primary oocyte (2n).
- The primary oocyte undergoes reduction division to form two haploid cells (n) of unequal size.
- The larger one is secondary oocyte (n) and the smaller one is first polar body (n).
- After ovulation the secondary oocyte undergoes equatorial division and it splits into two haploid cells of unequal size.

- The larger one is ovum (n) and the smaller one is second polar body (n).
- The nuclei of sperm (n) and ovum (n) then unite to form a diploid (2n) zygote.

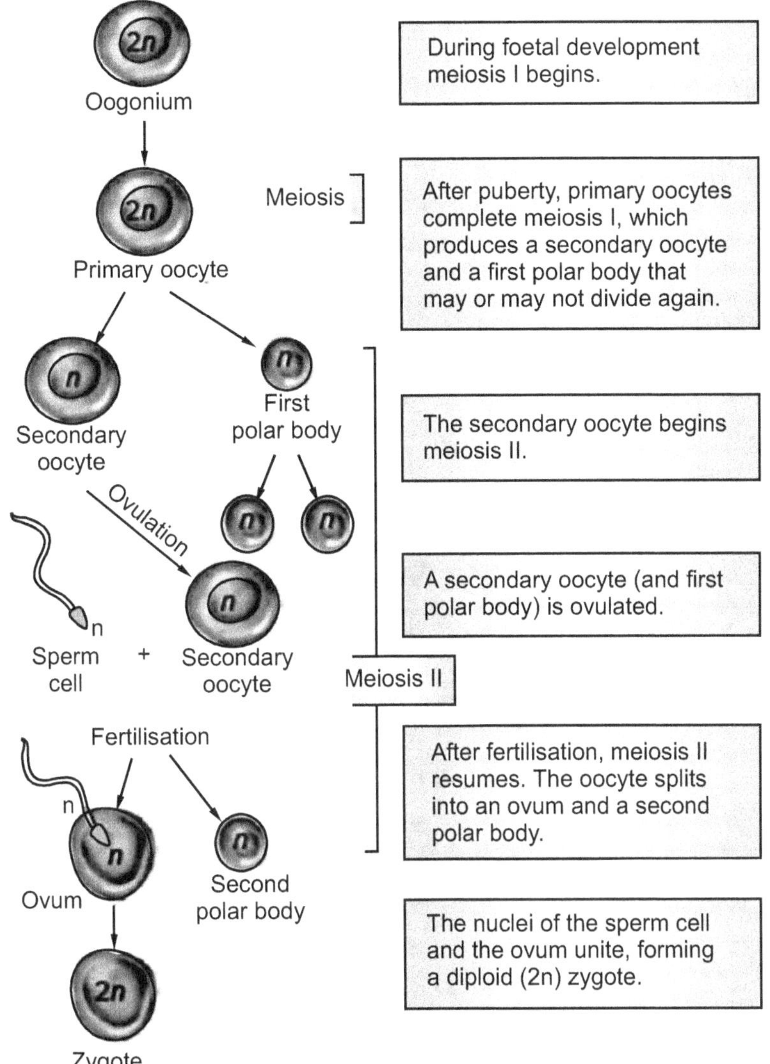

Fig. 7.10: Process of Oogenesis

7.4.3 Uterine Tubes (Fallopian Tubes)

- Females have two uterine tubes that extend laterally from the uterus.
- They are 10 cm long.
- They provide a route for sperm to reach an ovum and transport secondary oocytes and fertilise the ova from the ovaries to the uterus.
- It is divided into 3 parts:
  - ✓ **Infundibulum:** The funnel-shaped portion of each tube is called as infundibulum. It is close to ovary and is the open end of fallopian tubes. The infundibulum contains finger like projections called as fimbriae.

- ✓ **Ampulla:** It is the middle portion of the fallopian tube. It is the widest and longest portion; around two third the length of fallopian tube is ampulla.
- ✓ **Isthmus:** It is the last portion of the fallopian tubes. It is short, thick-walled, narrow portion of fallopian tubes, which joins the uterus.
- Histologically, the uterine tubes are composed of three layers,
  - ✓ **Mucosa:** It is the inner layer of uterine tube. It contains epithelium and lamina propria. The epithelium contains ciliated simple columnar cells, which helps to move the fertilised ovum (or secondary oocyte) along the uterine tube towards the uterus and nonciliated cells that have microvilli secrete a fluid that provides nutrition for ovum.
  - ✓ **Muscularis:** It is the middle layer of uterine tube. It consists of thick, circular rings of smooth muscles. Peristaltic contraction of muscularis and the ciliary contraction of mucosa help to move the oocytes or fertilized ovum towards the uterus.
  - ✓ **Serosa:** It is the outermost layer of uterine tube.

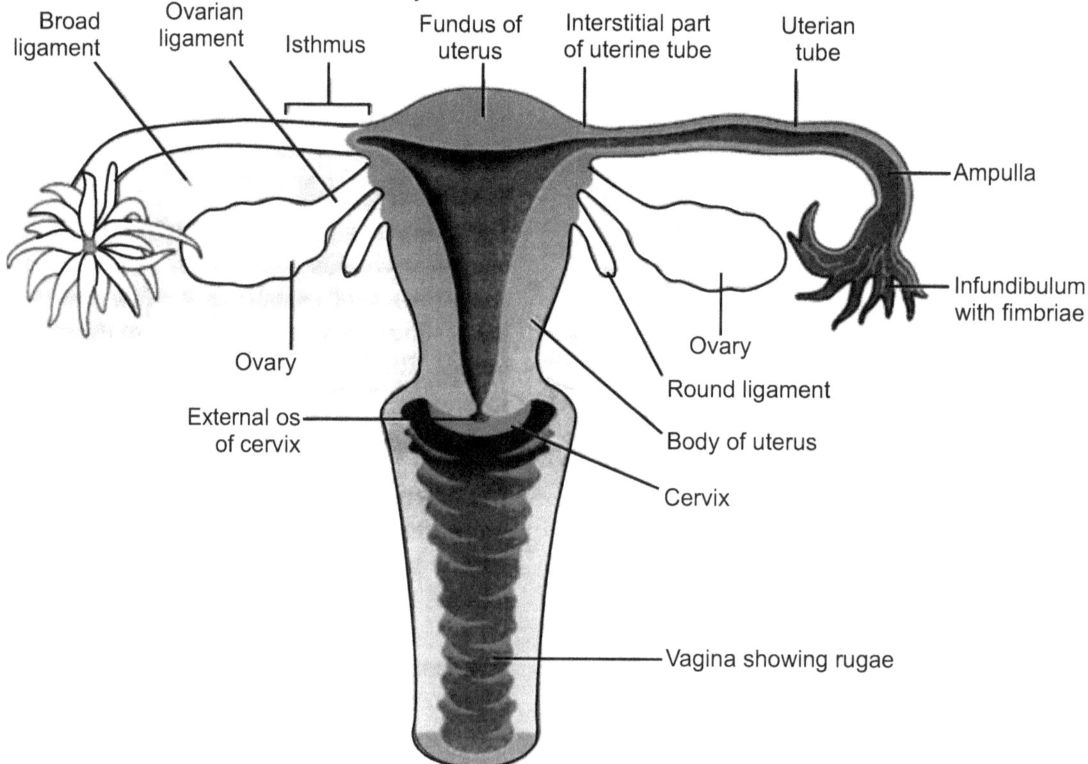

Fig. 7.11: Uterine tube

7.4.4 Uterus (Womb)

- It is situated between the urinary bladder and the rectum.
- It is a pear shaped organ.
- The non-pregnant uterus is around 7.5 cm long, 5 cm wide and 2.5 cm thick.

- It is the site of implantation of a fertilized ovum and development of the foetus during pregnancy.
- During reproductive cycles when implantation does not occur, the uterus is the source of menstrual flow.
- Histologically it is made up of three layers:
    - ✓ **Outer peritoneal layer**: Perimetrium
    - ✓ **Middle peritoneal layer:** Myometrium
    - ✓ **Inner peritoneal layer**: Endometrium
- The endometrium is further divided into two layers
    - ✓ **Stratum Functionalis:** It lines the uterus. During menstruation this layer sheds off.
    - ✓ **Stratum Basalis:** It is located below the stratum functionalis and it is a permanent layer.
- It divides into three parts
    - ✓ **Fundus:** It is a dome-shaped portion that lies superior to the uterine tubes.
    - ✓ **Body:** It is the tapering central portion.
    - ✓ **Cervix:** It is the inferior narrow portion that opens into the vagina.
- Between the uterus body and the cervix is the isthmus, a constricted region about 1 cm long.
- The inferior of the body of uterus is called as uterine cavity.

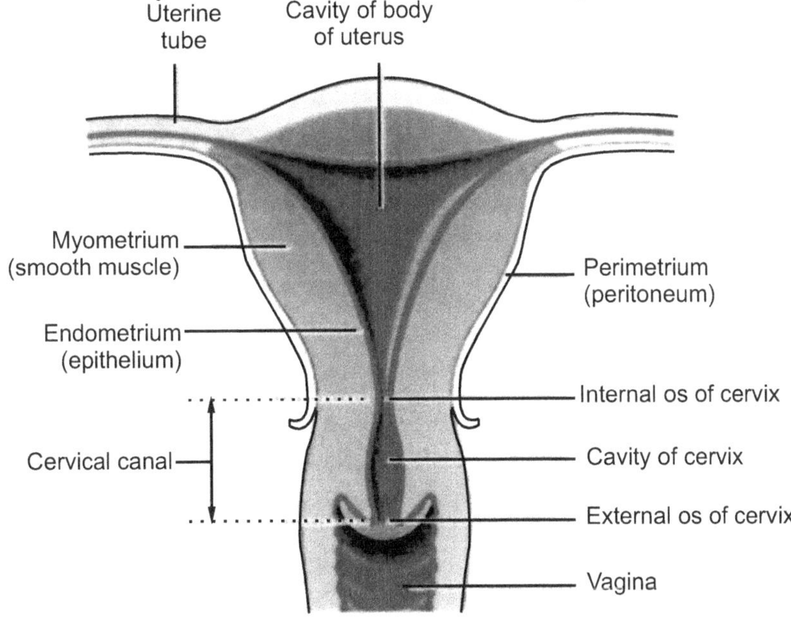

Fig. 7.12: Uterus

7.4.5 Vagina

- It is a tubular passage of about 10 cm long. fibromuscular canal that extends from the exterior of body to the uterine cervix.
- At the lower end vagina opens into cleft between the labia minora (Vestibule).

- In virgins this cleft is covered by a thin membrane called as hymen.
- Vagina serves as a passage way for the menstrual flow.
- It also receives semen from the penis during sexual intercourse.
- Vagina is situated between the urinary bladder and rectum.
- Vagina consists of three layers
  - ✓ Mucosa
  - ✓ Muscularis
  - ✓ Adventitia
- The mucosa consists of non-keratinised stratified squamous epithelium and areolar connective tissue that lies in a series of transverse folds called as rugae.
- The mucosa contains large stores of glycogen which on decomposition produce organic acids.
- The resulting acidic environment retards microbial growth but it is harmful to sperm.
- Alkaline components of semen, raises the pH of vagina and increases the viability of sperm.
- Muscularis layer is composed of outer circular layers and inner longitudinal layer of smooth muscles.
- Adventitia is the superficial layer of vagina.

7.4.6 External Organs of the Female Reproductive System

Vulva (Pudendum)

- It is the external genital of female.
- It consists of following components;
  - ✓ **Mons pubis:** Anterior to the vaginal and urethral opening is the mons penis, an elevation of the adipose tissue covered by skin and coarse pubic hair that cushions the pubic symphysis of skin called as labia majora. It is covered by pubic hair and contains an abundance of adipose tissue, oil glands and sweat glands.
  - ✓ **Labia minora:** Medial to the labia majora is two smaller folds of skin called as labia minora. They do not contain fatty tissue and hair.
  - ✓ **Clitoris:** It is a small, cylindrical mass of erectile tissue and nerves. It is located at anterior junction of labia minora. The clitoris is homologous to penis and enlarges on excitation.

Vestibule

- It is the region between labia minora.
- The vaginal orifice is the opening of vagina to the exterior and is bordered by the hymen.
- External urethral orifice is the opening of the urethra to the exterior.
- The Bartholin's glands are present on either side of vaginal orifice and produce a small quantity of mucus during sexual arousal and intercourse.

Bulb of the vestibule

- It consists of two elongated masses of erectile tissue just deep to the labia on either side of the vaginal orifice
- The bulb of the vestibule is homologous to the corpus spongiosum and bulb of the penis in males.

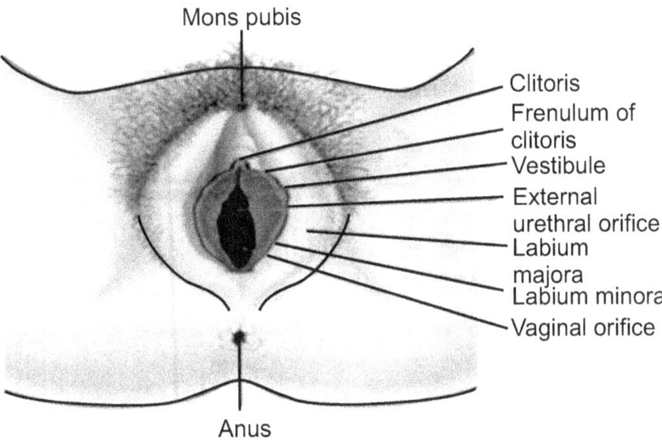

Fig. 7.13: Vulva

7.5 FEMALE REPRODUCTIVE CYCLE (MENSTRUAL CYCLE)

- Consider the menstrual cycle of 28 days.
- It consists of 4 phases:
  - ✓ Menstrual phase
  - ✓ Preovulatory phase
  - ✓ Ovulation phase
  - ✓ Postovulatory phase

Menstrual Phase

- It is also called as menstruation or mense.
- It lasts for first five days of cycle.
- Menstrual flow from the uterus consists of 50-150 ml of blood, tissue fluid, mucus and epithelial cells shed from the endometrium.
- This discharge occurs because the declining levels of progesterone and estrogen stimulate the release of prostaglandins that causes the constriction of arteries of uterus.
- This leads to ischemic condition of epithelial cells of endometrium and they start to die.
- The dead endometrium (stratum functionalis) is removed and only stratum basalis which is very thin is left adhered to the uterus.
- Menstrual flow passes from uterine cavity through the vagina to the exterior.

Preovulatory Phase

- The preovulatory phase is the time between the end of menstruation and ovulation.
- It lasts for 6-12 days.

- The growing ovarian follicle liberates estrogens into blood.
- The follicles stimulate the repair of endometrium.
- The cells of stratum basalis undergo mitosis and produce a new stratum functionalis.
- The thickness of endometrium approximately doubles to about 4-10 mm.
- The preovulatory phase is called as proliferative phase because the endometrium is proliferating.

Ovulation Phase

- Ovulation is the rupture of mature (graafian) follicle and the release of secondary oocytes into the pelvic cavity.
- It occurs on 14th day of cycle.
- If fertilization does not occur within 24 hours of ovulation then the egg degenerates.
- The small amount of blood that leaks into the pelvic cavity from the ruptured follicle can cause pain known as mittelschmerz.

Postovulatory Phase

- The time between ovulation and the onset of next menses is called as postovulatory phases.
- It lasts for 14 days from 16 to 28 days.
- Progesterone and estrogen produced by corpus luteum promotes growth and coiling of the endometrium and thickening of endometrium to 12-18 mm.
- The endometrial glands secrete glycogen.
- All these are preovulatory changes for implantation of fertilized ovum lasts for one week.
- If the ovum is not fertilized, the corpus luteum gets converted to corpus albicans and the secretion of estrogen and progesterone is stopped, leading to menstruation.

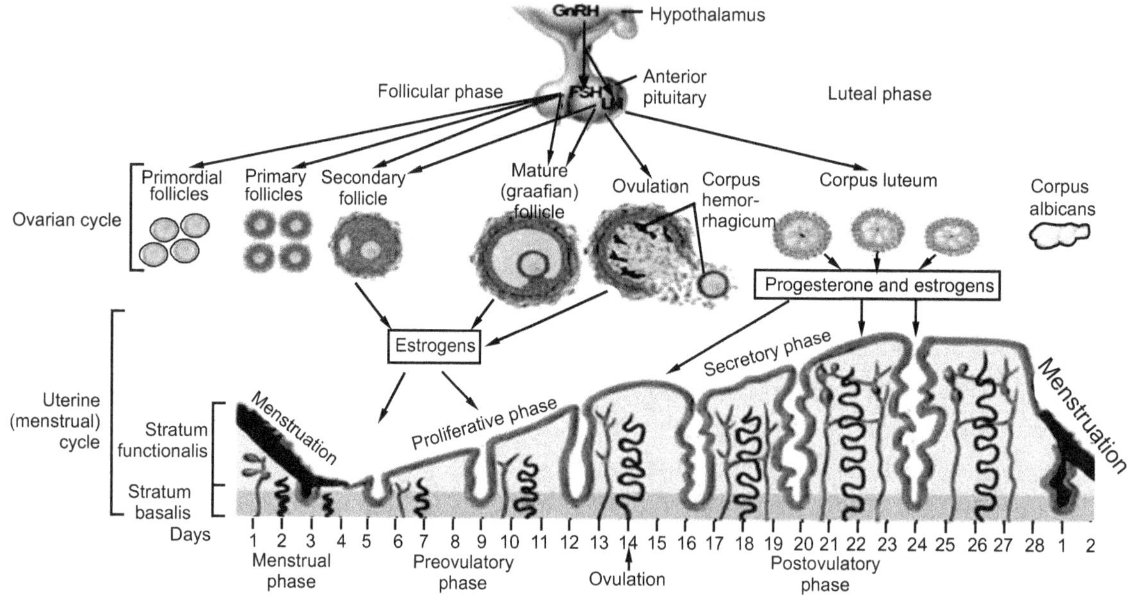

Fig. 7.14: Female reproductive cycle

7.6 BREAST (MAMMARY GLANDS)

- These are the accessory glands of the female reproductive system.
- Each breast has one pigmented projection called as nipple consisting of closely spaced openings of ducts called as lactiferous ducts, where milk emerges.
- The circular pigmented area around the nipple is called as areolar. It appears rough because it contains modified sebaceous glands.
- Each breast consists of 15-20 lobes separated by variable amount of adipose tissue.
- Each lobe is made up of several smaller compartments called as lobules, composed of grape like cluster of milk secreting glands called as alveoli.
- The alveoli secrete milk into the secondary lobules and then into mammary ducts.
- Near the nipple, the mammary ducts expand to form sinuses called as lactiferous sinuses where milk is stored before draining into a lactiferous duct.
- Each lactiferous duct carries milk from one of the lobe to the exterior.

Functions

- Synthesis, secretion and ejection of milk is called as lactation.
- Milk production is stimulated by prolactin hormone secreted by anterior pituitary.

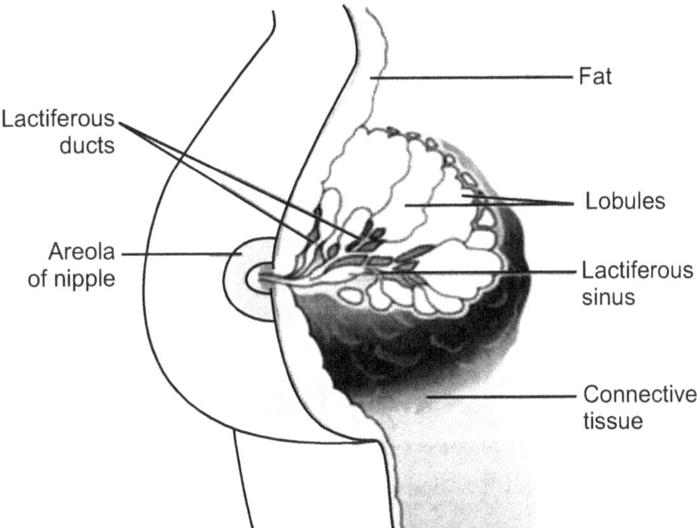

Fig. 7.15: Mammary gland

7.7 PREGNANCY AND PARTURITION

- Pregnancy is a sequence of events that includes fertilization, implantation, embryonic development (first 8 weeks), fetal development (9 month till birth) and parturition.

Fertilization:

- A secondary oocyte is visible for about 24 hours after ovulation, whereas the sperms remain viable in the vagina for about 48 hours after ejaculation.
- For fertilization to occur, sexual intercourse must occur between a 3 day windows that is from 2 days before ovulation to 1 day after ovulation.

- The process leading to fertilization begins when the sperm cells swim upwards through the vagina and uterine tube by movements of their tails.
- Although hundreds of sperms surround the ovum and undergo acrosome reaction (i.e. release the enzymes to penetrate the ovum), only the first sperm cell to penetrate the plasma membrane of the ovum fuses with it to procures a fertilized ovum or zygote.
- This process is called as fertilization and it normally occurs in the upper portion of the uterine tube.
- The time span from fertilization to birth is termed as the gestation period.
- As the zygote moves down the uterine tube towards the uterine cavity, it undergoes a series of rapid mitotic division, resulting in a hollow ball like mass of cells called as blastula or blastocyst.
- The blastocyst has an outer covering of cells called the trophoblast, an inner cell mass and an internal fluid filled cavity called as blastocele.

Implantation:

- About 6 days after fertilization, the blastocyst attaches to the endometrial lining of the uterus and eventually gets embedded in it, a process called as implantation.
- At this stage, the trophoblast secretes human chorionic gonadotropin hormone (hCG), whose action are similar to those of luteinizing hormone.
- hCG prevents the degeneration of corpus luteum and sustains in secretion of progesterone and estrogen, thereby preventing menstruation.

Labor or Parturition:

- It is the process by which the fetus is expelled from the uterus through the vagina. It is also known as parturition.
- The onset of labour is associated with several placental and fetal hormones.
- The progesterone inhibits the uterine contractions and labor cannot take place until its effects are diminished.
- Toward the end of gestation period, the levels of estrogens rise sharply, producing changes that overcome the inhibiting effects of progesterone.
- The rise in estrogens level results into secretion of adrenocorticotropic hormone from the fetal adrenal gland.
- Also they secrete cortisol and dehydroepiandrosterone, the major adrenal androgen.
- The placental tissue converts dehydroepiandrosterone into an estrogen.
- High levels of estrogens hormone causes release of oxytocin by the posterior pituitary gland that stimulates the uterine contractions and relaxin that helps in dilatation of uterine cervix.
- Uterine contractions occur in waves that start at the top of uterus and move downward, eventually expelling the fetus.
- True labour begins when uterine contractions occur at regular intervals, usually producing pain.

- Another symptom of true labour in some women is localization of pain in the back that is amplified by walking.
- The most reliable indicator of true labour is dilation of cervix and a discharge of blood-containing mucus into the cervical canal.
- True labour can be divided into three stages;

Stage of dilation:

- It is the time from the onset of labour to the complete dilation of cervix.
- It typically lasts 6-12 hours.
- It is characterised by regular contractions of the uterus, usually a rupturing of amniotic sac and complete dilation (up to 10 cm) of the cervix.

Stage of expulsion:

- The time (10 minutes to several hours) from complete cervical dilation to delivery of the baby is the stage of expulsion.

Placental stage:

- The time (5-30 minutes or more) after delivery until the placenta is expelled by powerful uterine contractions is the placental stage.
- These contractions also constrict the blood vessels that were torn during delivery, reducing the likelihood of hemorrhage.

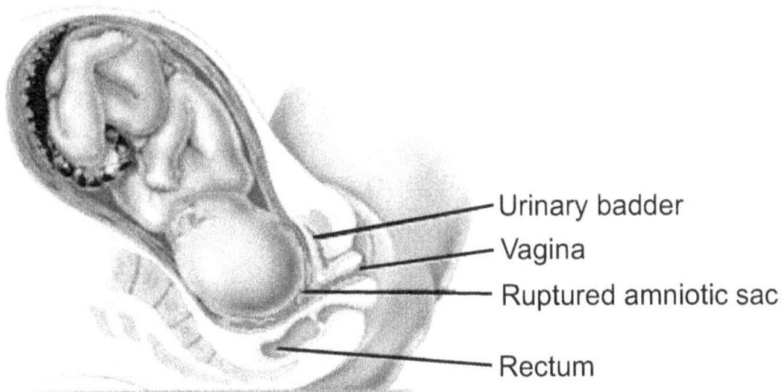

Stage of dilation

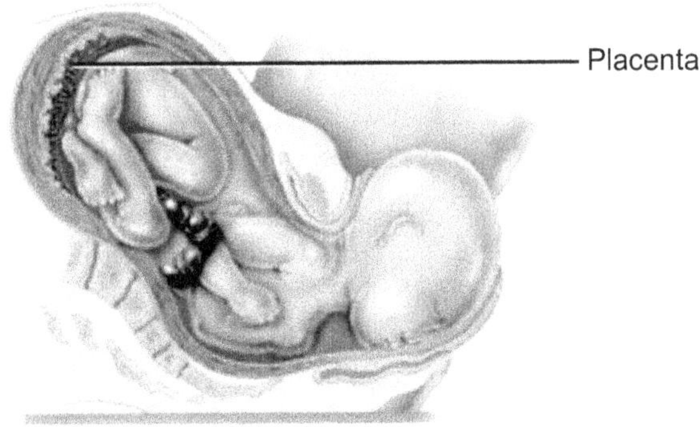

Stage of expulsion

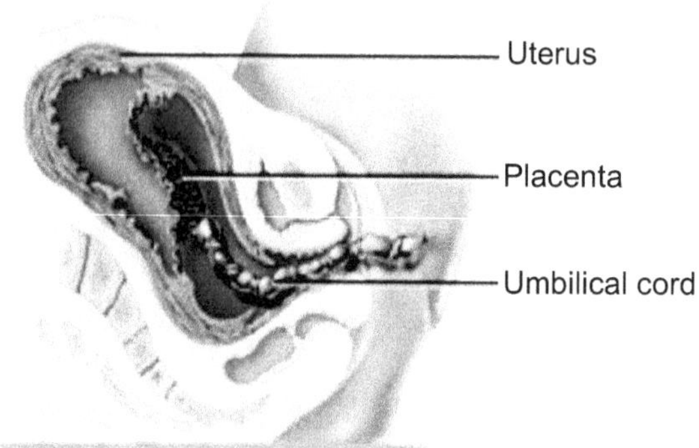

Placental stage

Fig. 7.16: Different stages of labour

7.8 DISORDERS OF THE REPRODUCTIVE SYSTEM

Testicular cancer

- It is common in males between the ages of 20-35 years.
- More than 95% of testicular cancer arises from spermatogonia within the seminiferous tubules.
- The early sign of testicular cancer is a mass in the testis associated with a sensation of testicular heaviness in the lower abdomen.

Prostrate cancer

- The symptoms are fever, chills, frequent urination, difficulty in urinating, burning or painful urination, low back pain, joint and muscle pain, blood in the urine, or painful ejaculation.
- There are two main types of prostatis
    ✓ **Acute prostatitis:** Prostrate becomes swollen for short term.
    ✓ **Chronic prostatitis:** Long term inflammation of prostrate.

Endometriosis

- It is characterised by the growth of endometrial tissue outside the uterus.
- The symptoms include premenstrual pain or usually severe menstrual pain, pain in lower abdomen and pelvic area and reduced fertility.

Breast cancer

- The first sign of breast cancer is a breast lump.
- Mammography is the most effective technique in detecting the tumour.
- The stages range from early curable breast cancer to metastatic breast cancer
- The treatment for breast cancer may include hormone therapy, chemotherapy, radiation therapy or combination of this therapy.

Ovarian cancer

- It is the carcinoma of ovaries.
- The symptoms include abdominal discomfort, heart burn, nausea, loss of appetite, bloating and flatulence.

- The symptom includes enlarged abdomen, abdominal-pelvic pain, urinary complications, menstrual irregularities and heavy menstrual bleeding.

Cervical cancer

- It is the carcinoma of cervix of uterus
- It starts with cervical dysplasia, a change in the shape, growth and number of cervical cells.
- The symptoms are vaginal bleeding, contact bleeding or a vaginal mass may indicate the presence of malignancy, moderate pain during sexual intercourse and vaginal discharge.

Vulvovaginal candidiasis

- *Candia albicans* is yeast like fungus that commonly grows on mucus of gastrointestinal tract and genitourinary tracts.
- It is characterised by inflammation of vagina, severe itching, a thick, yellow, cheesy discharge, yeasty odour and pain.

Chlamydia

- It is a sexually transmitted disease caused by bacterium *Chlamydia trachomatis*.
- The initial infection is asymptomatic and thus difficult to detect clinically.
- In males, urethritis is the principal result, causing a clear discharge, burning sensation during urination, frequent urination and painful urination.

Syphilis

- It is caused by the bacterium *Treponema pallidum*
- It is transmitted through sexual contact or exchange of blood, or through the placenta to the foetus.
- The disease progresses through several stages.
- During the primary stage, a painless open sore, called a chancre develops at the point of contact.
- The chancre heals within 1 to 5 weeks.
- From 6 to 24 weeks later, the signs and symptoms such as a skin rash, fever and aches in the joints appear.
- The symptoms of secondary stage are systemic and the infection spreads to all major body parts.
- When signs of organ degeneration appear, the disease is said to be in the tertiary stage.
- If the nervous system is involved, the tertiary stage is called neurosyphilis.

Genital herpes

- It is an incurable sexually transmitted disease.
- Type II herpes simplex virus (HSV-2) causes genital infections, producing painful blisters on the prepuce, glans penis and penile shaft in males and on the vulva or sometimes high up in the vagina in females.

QUESTIONS

Short Answer Questions:

1. Discuss the hormonal control of testes.
2. Write a note on sperm.
3. Enlist and define any three STDs.
4. Write a note on ovaries.
5. Explain oogenesis process.
6. Draw a neat labelled diagram of ovary representing various stages of follicles.
7. Explain the structure of sperm and process of spermatogenesis.
8. Draw neat diagram of menstrual cycle.

Long Answer Questions:

1. Write a note on female reproductive cycle.
2. Enlist the different parts of male reproductive system and give its anatomy and physiology.
3. Explain the process of oogenesis and follicular development.
4. Explain in detail various phases of menstrual cycle.
5. Draw neat labelled diagram of female reproductive organs in the pelvis. Explain menstrual cycle with hormonal changes.
6. Explain the process of pregnancy and different stages of labour.

Chapter 8

INTRODUCTION TO GENETICS

♦ LEARNING OBJECTIVES ♦

❖ To study the structure of chromosome and gene.

❖ To describe the structure of DNA.

❖ To study the steps of protein synthesis.

8.1 CHROMOSOMES

- These are thread-like structures located inside the nucleus of animal and plant cells.

- Chromosomes are passed on from parents to offspring.

- The term chromosome is derived from a Greek word 'chroma' means 'colour' and 'soma' means 'body'.

- The chromosomes are named so because they are cellular structures or cellular bodies and they are strongly stained by some dyes used in research.

- Chromosomes are organized structure of DNA and proteins found in the cells.

- Chromosomes are made up of proteins and a molecule of deoxyribonucleic acid (DNA).

- Human being have 23 pairs of chromosomes.

- Chromosomes carry all the information that help a cell grows, survive and reproduce.

- DNA segments with specific patterns are called as genes.

- The chromosomes are found in the nucleus of the cell.

- In prokaryotic organisms, the DNA is not present in the nucleus; the DNA floats in the cytoplasm in area called as nucleoid.

- The chromosomes vary widely between different organisms.

- Eukaryotic cells have large number of linear chromosomes and cells of prokaryotes have smaller and circular DNA.

- Cells may contain more than one type of chromosome, like in most eukaryotic cells, the mitochondria and the chloroplasts in plant cells possess their own set of chromosomes.

- In nucleus of eukaryotic organism, the chromosomes are packed by proteins to form a compact structure called as chromatin.

- This condensation allows long molecules of DNA to fit into the cell nucleus.
- Chromosomes are more condensed then the chromatin and they are essential for cell division.
- The chromosomes are replicated, divided and passed on to the daughter cells, to ensure genetic diversity and survival of the progeny.
- Duplicated chromosomes contain two identical copies known as chromtids or sister chromatids, they are joined by a centromere.
- Compaction of the chromosomes during the cell division process results in the four-arm structure.
- Recombination of chromosome plays a vital role in the genetic diversity.
- Incorrect multiplication of the chromosomes may lead to mitotic failure or death of the cell, it may lead to apoptosis and sometimes may be cancerous.
- Chromosomes play an important role that ensures DNA is copied and distributed accurately in the process of cell division.

8.2 CHROMOSOME STRUCTURE

- In eukarytoic cells, chromosomes are composed of single molecule of DNA with many copies of five types of histones.
- Histones are proteins molecules and are rich in lysine and arginine residues, they are positively charged.
- Hence, they bind tightly to the negatively charged phosphates in the DNA sequence.
- A small number of non-histone proteins are also present, these are mostly transcription factors.
- Transcription factors regulate the parts of DNA to be transcribed into RNA.
- During most of the cell's life cycle, chromosomes are elongated and cannot be observed under the microscope.
- During the S phase of mitotic cell cycle the chromosomes are duplicated.
- At the beginning of mitosis the chromosomes are duplicated and they begin to condense into short structures which can be stained and observed easily under the light microscope.
- These duplicated condensed chromosomes are known as dyads.
- The duplicated chromosomes are held together at the region of centromeres.
- The centromeres in humans are made of about 1-10 million base pairs of DNA.
- The DNA of the centromere are mostly repetitive short sequences of DNA, the sequences are repeated over and over in tandem arrays.
- The attached, duplicated chromosomes are commonly called as sister chromatids.
- Kinetochores are the attachment point for spindle fibers which helps to pull apart the sister chromatids as the mitosis process proceeds to anaphase stage.
- The kinetochores are a complex of about 80 different proteins.
- The shorter arm of two arms of the chromosome extending from the centromere is called the p arm and the longer arm is known the q arm.

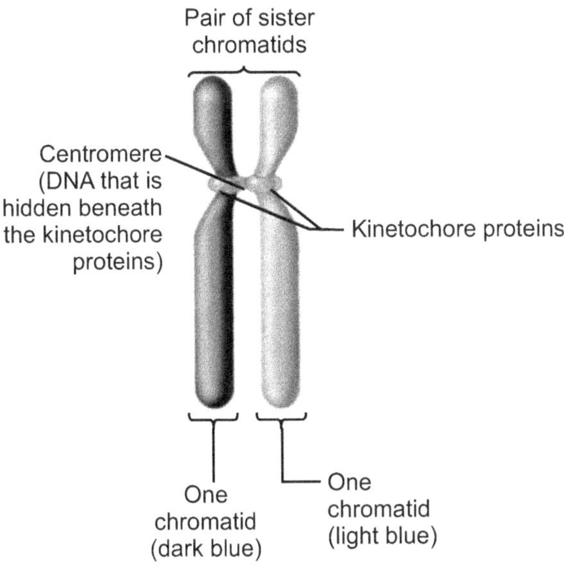

Fig. 8.1: Structure of Chromosome

Human Chromosomes

- Humans chromosomes are of two types autosomes and sex chromosomes.
- Genetic traits that are linked to the sex of the person are passed on through the sex chromosomes.
- The rest of the genetic information is present in the autosomes.
- Humans have 23 pairs of chromosomes in their cells, of which 22 pairs are autosomes and one pair of sex chromosomes, making a total of 46 chromosomes in each cell.
- Many copies of mitochondrial genome are present in human cells.

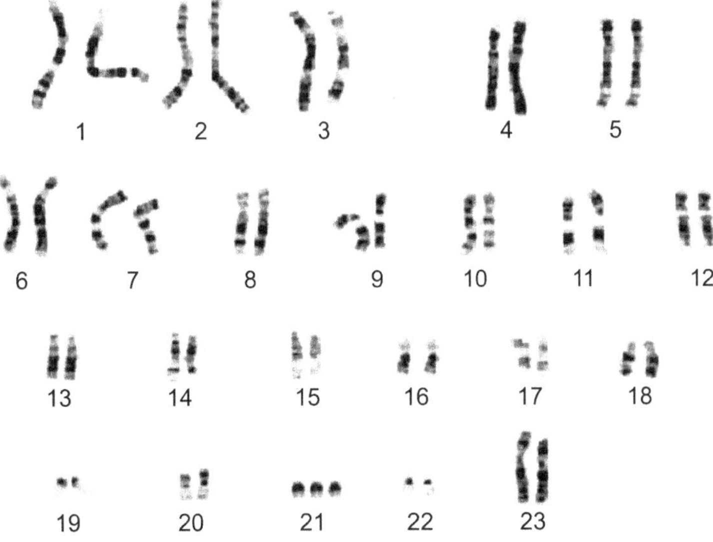

Fig. 8.2: Structure of Chromosome in human

Sex Chromosomes

- Sex chromosomes differ in form of size, behaviour from the ordinary chromosome.
- The sex chromosomes determine the sex of an individual during reproduction.
- These sex chromosomes differ between the male and the females.
- Females have two copies of X chromosome, males have one X chromosome and one Y chromosome.
- In the process of sexual reproduction in humans, two different gametes fuse to form a zygote.

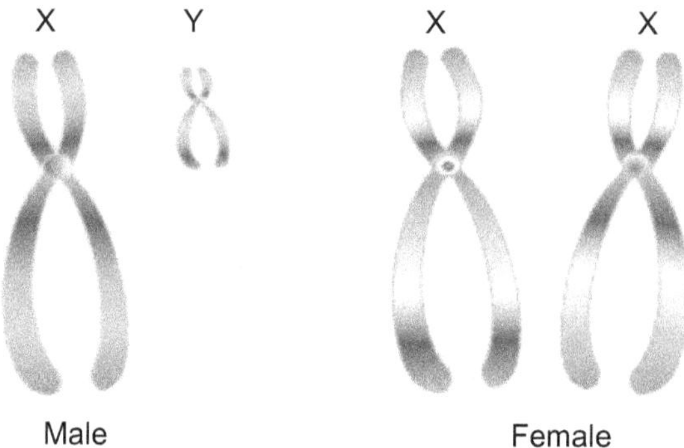

Fig. 8.3: Structure of Sex Chromosome

Function of Chromosomes

Functions of chromosomes are as follows:

- **Genetic Code Storage:** Chromosome contains the genetic material that is required by the organism to develop and grow. DNA molecules are made of chain of units called as genes. Genes are those sections of the DNA which code for specific proteins required by the cell for its proper functioning.
- **Sex Determination:** Humans have 23 pairs of chromosomes out of which one pair is the sex chromosome. Females have two X chromosomes and males have one X and one Y chromosome. The sex of the child is determined by the chromosome passed down by the male. If X chromosome is passed out of XY chromosome, the child will be a female and if a Y chromosome is passed, a male child develops.
- **Control of Cell Division:** Chromosomes check successful division of cells during the process of mitosis. The chromosomes of the parent cells insure that the correct information is passed on to the daughter cells required by the cell to grow and develop correctly.
- **Formation of Proteins and Storage:** Proteins are essential for the activity of a cell. The chromosomes direct the sequences of proteins formed in our body and also maintain the order of DNA. The proteins are also stored in the coiled structure of the chromosomes. These proteins bound to the DNA help in proper packaging of the DNA.

Genes:

- Genes are made of a substance called as deoxyribonucleic acid (DNA).
- They give instructions for a living being to make molecules called as proteins.

- Genes are a section of DNA that are incharge of different functions like making proteins.
- Long strands of DNA with lots of genes make up chromosomes.
- DNA molecules are found in the chromosomes.
- Chromosomes are located inside of the nucleus of cells.
- Each chromosome is one long single molecule of DNA. This DNA contains important genetic information.
- Chromosomes have a unique structure, which helps to keep the DNA tightly wrapped around the proteins called as histones.
- If the DNA molecules were not bound by the histones, they would be too long to fit inside of the cell.
- Genes vary in complexity. In humans, they range in size from a few hundred DNA bases to more than 2 million bases.
- Different living things have different shapes and numbers of chromosomes.
- Humans have 23 pairs of chromosomes, or a total of 46.
- DNA contains the biological instructions that make each species unique.
- DNA is passed from an adult organisms to their offspring during reproduction.
- The building blocks of DNA are called as nucleotides.
- Nucleotides have three parts: A phosphate group, a sugar group and one of four types of nitrogen bases.
- A gene consists of a long combination of four different nucleotide bases, or chemicals.
- There are many possible combinations.
- The four nucleotides are:
  o A (adenine)
  o C (cytosine)
  o G (guanine)
  o T (thymine)
- Different combinations of the letters ACGT give people different characteristics.
- For example, a person with the combination ATCGTT may have blue eyes, while somebody with the combination ATCGCT may have brown eyes.
- Genes carry the codes ACGT.
- Each person has thousands of genes.
- They are like a computer program, and they make the individual what they are.
- A gene is a tiny section of a long DNA double helix molecule, which consists of a linear sequence of base pairs.
- A gene is any section along the DNA with instructions encoded that allow a cell to produce a specific product - usually a protein, such as an enzyme - that triggers one precise action.
- DNA is the chemical that appears in strands.

- Every cell in a person's body has the same DNA, but each person's DNA is different. This is what makes each person unique.
- DNA is made up of two long-paired strands spiraled into the famous double helix.
- Each strand contains millions of chemical building blocks called as bases.

Function

- Genes decide almost everything about a living being. One or more genes can affect a specific trait. Genes may interact with an individual's environment too and change what the gene makes.
- Genes affect hundreds of internal and external factors, such as whether a person will get a particular colour of eyes or what diseases they may develop.
- Some diseases, such as Sickle-cell anemia and Huntington's disease are inherited and these are also affected by genes.

Deoxy-ribonucleic acid (DNA)

- Deoxyribonucleic acid is a molecule composed of two chains that coil around each other to form a double helix carrying the genetic instructions used in the growth, development, functioning and reproduction of all known living organisms and many viruses.
- DNA was first isolated by Friedrich Miescher in 1869.
- Its molecular structure was first identified by Francis Crick and James Watson at the Cavendish Laboratory within the University of Cambridge in 1953, whose model-building efforts were guided by X-ray diffraction data acquired by Raymond Gosling, who was a post-graduate student of Rosalind Franklin.
- DNA and ribonucleic acid (RNA) are nucleic acids; alongside proteins, lipids and complex carbohydrates (polysaccharides), nucleic acids are one of the four major types of macromolecules that are essential for all known forms of life.
- The two DNA strands are also known as polynucleotides as they are composed of simpler monomeric units called as nucleotides.
- Each nucleotide is composed of one of four nitrogen-containing nucleobases (cytosine [C], guanine [G], adenine [A] or thymine [T]), a sugar called deoxyribose, and a phosphate group.
- The nucleotides are joined to one another in a chain by covalent bonds between the sugar of one nucleotide and the phosphate of the next, resulting in an alternating sugar-phosphate backbone.
- The nitrogenous bases of the two separate polynucleotide strands are bound together, according to base pairing rules (A with T and C with G), with hydrogen bonds to make double-stranded DNA.
- The complementary nitrogenous bases are divided into two groups, pyrimidines and purines.
- In DNA, the pyrimidines are thymine and cytosine; the purines are adenine and guanine.

- Both strands of double-stranded DNA store the same biological information.

- This information is replicated as and when the two strands separate.

- A large part of DNA (more than 98% for humans) is non-coding, meaning that these sections do not serve as patterns for protein sequences.

- The two strands of DNA run in opposite directions to each other and are thus antiparallel.

- Attached to each sugar is one of four types of nucleobases (informally, bases).

- It is the sequence of these four nucleobases along the backbone that encodes genetic information.

- RNA strands are created using DNA strands as a template in a process called as transcription.

- Under the genetic code, these RNA strands specify the sequence of amino acids within proteins in a process called as translation.

- The DNA molecule has two important properties.

- **It can make copies of itself**. If you pull the two strands apart, each can be used to make the other one (and a new DNA molecule).

- **It can carry information**. The order of the bases along a strand is a code - a code for making proteins.

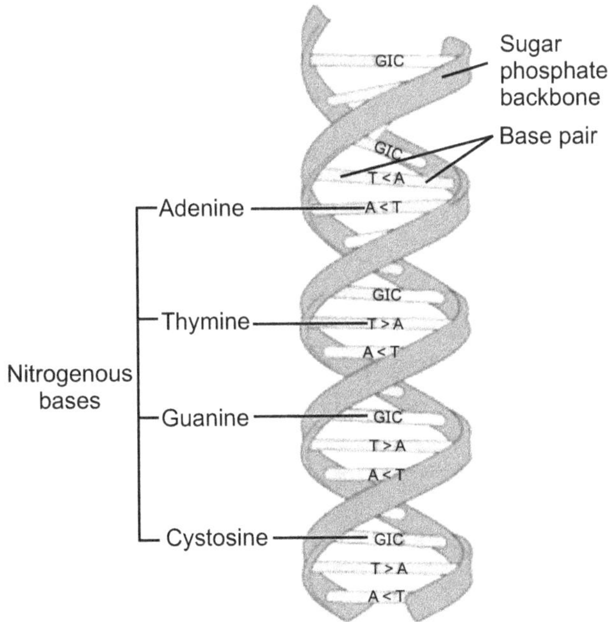

Fig. 8.4: Double helix struture of DNA

8.3 PROTEIN SYNTHESIS

- The proteins are responsible for determination of physical and chemical characteristics of cells and organisms.
- Some proteins help in assembling cellular structures such as the plasma membrane, the cytoskeleton and other organelles.
- Others proteins serve as hormones, antibodies and contractile elements in muscular tissue, enzymes regulating the rates of the numerous chemical reactions, carrying various materials in the blood.
- **Genome:** All the genes in an organism.
- **Proteome:** All the proteins in an organism.

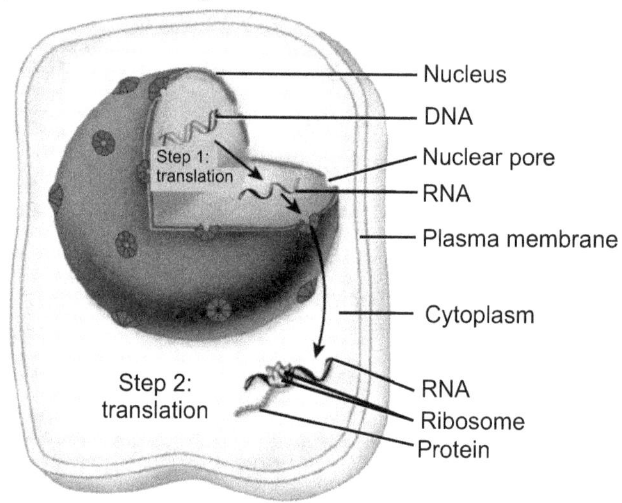

Fig. 8.5: Protein synthesis

Protein Synthesis:
- A gene's DNA is used as a template for synthesis of a specific protein.
- **Transcription:** The information encoded in a specific region of DNA is transcribed (copied) to produce a specific molecule of RNA (ribonucleic acid).
- **Translation:** The RNA attaches to a ribosome, where the information contained in RNA is translated into a corresponding sequence of amino acids to form a new protein molecule.
- DNA and RNA store genetic information as sets of three nucleotides.
- A sequence of three nucleotides in DNA is called a base triplet.
- Each DNA base triplet is transcribed as a complementary sequence of three nucleotides, called a codon.
- A given codon specifies a particular amino acid.

Transcription:
- Transcription is the first stage of the expression of genes into proteins.
- In transcription, a mRNA (messenger RNA) intermediate is transcribed from one of the strands of the DNA molecule.

- The RNA is called as messenger RNA because it carries the 'message' or genetic information from the DNA to the ribosomes, where the information is used to make proteins.
- The process of transcription occurs in the nucleus.
- In this process the genetic information represented by the sequence of base triplets in DNA serves as a template for copying the information into a complementary sequence of codons.
- Three types of RNA are made from the DNA template:
  - **Messenger RNA (mRNA):** It directs the synthesis of a protein.
  - **Ribosomal RNA (rRNA):** It joins with ribosomal proteins to make ribosomes.
  - **Transfer RNA (tRNA):** It binds to an amino acid and holds it in place on a ribosome until it is incorporated into a protein during translation.
- Transcription may be broken into four stages:
  - ✓ Initiation
  - ✓ Elongation
  - ✓ Termination
  - ✓ Processing
- **Initiation:** The DNA molecule unwinds and separates to form a small open complex. RNA polymerase binds to the promoter of the template strand.
- **Elongation:** RNA polymerase moves along the template strand, synthesising an mRNA molecule. In prokaryotes RNA polymerase is a holoenzyme consisting of a number of subunits, including a sigma factor (transcription factor) that recognises the promoter. In eukaryotes there are three RNA polymerases: I, II and III. The process includes a proofreading mechanism.
- **Termination:** In prokaryotes there are two ways in which transcription is terminated. In Rho-dependent termination, a protein factor called "Rho" is responsible for disrupting the complex involving the template strand, RNA polymerase and RNA molecule. In Rho-independent termination, a loop forms at the end of the RNA molecule, causing it to detach itself. Termination in eukaryotes is more complicated, involving the addition of additional adenine nucleotides at the 3' of the RNA transcript (a process referred to as polyadenylation).
- **Processing:** After transcription the RNA molecule is processed in a number of ways: introns are removed and the exons are spliced together to form a mature mRNA molecule consisting of a single protein-coding sequence. RNA synthesis involves the normal base pairing rules, but the base thymine is replaced with the base uracil.
- One end of the tRNA carries a specific amino acid, and the opposite end consists of a triplet of nucleotides called an anticodon.
- The enzyme RNA polymerase catalyzes transcription of DNA.
- The segment of DNA where transcription begins, a special nucleotide sequence called a promoter, is located near the beginning of a gene where RNA polymerase attaches to the DNA.

- During transcription, bases pair in a complementary manner: The bases cytosine (C), guanine (G), and thymine (T) in the DNA template pair with guanine, cytosine, and adenine (A), respectively, in the RNA strand.

- However, adenine in the DNA template pairs with uracil (U), not thymine, in RNA.

- Transcription of the DNA strand ends at another special nucleotide sequence called a terminator, which specifies the end of the gene.

- When RNA polymerase reaches the terminator, the enzyme detaches from the transcribed RNA molecule and the DNA strand.

- The resulting product is a functional mRNA molecule that passes through a pore in the nuclear envelope to reach the cytoplasm, where translation takes place.

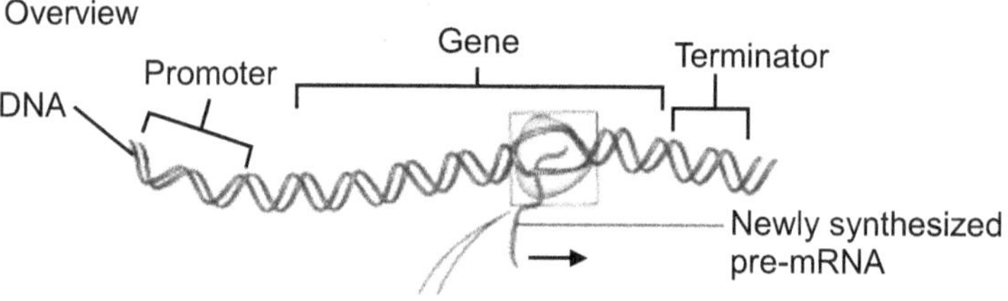

Fig. 8.6: Transcription Process

Translation:

- Translation is the process in which cellular ribosomes create proteins.

- In translation, messenger RNA (mRNA) produced by transcription is decoded by a ribosome complex to produce a specific amino acid chain, or polypeptide, that will later fold into an active protein.

- Translation occurs in the cells cytoplasm, where the large and small subunits of the ribosome are located, and bind to the mRNA.

- The ribosome facilitates decoding by inducing the binding of tRNAs with complementary anticodon sequences to that of the mRNA.

- The tRNAs carry specific amino acids that are chained together into a polypeptide as the mRNA passes through and is read by the ribosome.

- Translation proceeds in four phases:
  - ✓ Initiation
  - ✓ Elongation
  - ✓ Translocation
  - ✓ Termination

- **Initiation:** The small subunit of the ribosome binds at the 5' end of the mRNA molecule and moves in a 3' direction until it meets a start codon (AUG). It then forms a complex with the large unit of the ribosome complex and an initiation tRNA molecule.

- **Elongation:** Subsequent codons on the mRNA molecule determine which tRNA molecule linked to an amino acid binds to the mRNA. An enzyme peptidyl transferase links the amino acids together using peptide bonds. The process continues, producing a chain of amino acids as the ribosome moves along the mRNA molecule.

- **Termination:** Translation in terminated when the ribosomal complex reached one or more stop codons (UAA, UAG, UGA). The ribosomal complex in eukaryotes is larger and more complicated than in prokaryotes. In addition, the processes of transcription and translation are divided in eukaryotes between the nucleus (transcription) and the cytoplasm (translation), which provides more opportunities for the regulation of gene expression.
- The small subunit of a ribosome has a binding site for mRNA; the large subunit has two binding sites for tRNA molecules, a P site and an A site
- The first tRNA molecule bearing its specific amino acid attaches to mRNA at the P site.
- The A site holds the next tRNA molecule bearing its amino acid.

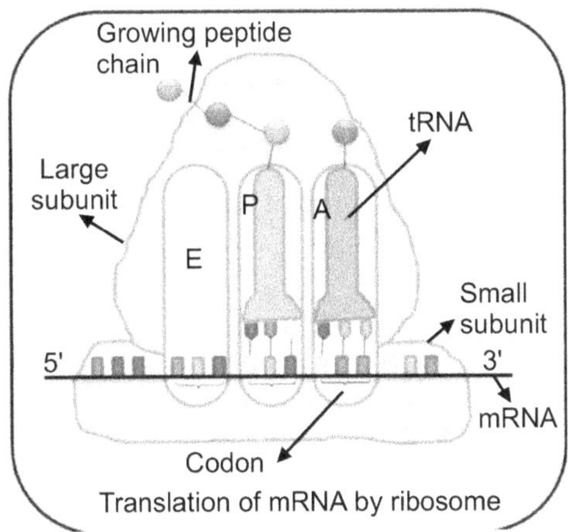

Fig. 8.7: Translation process

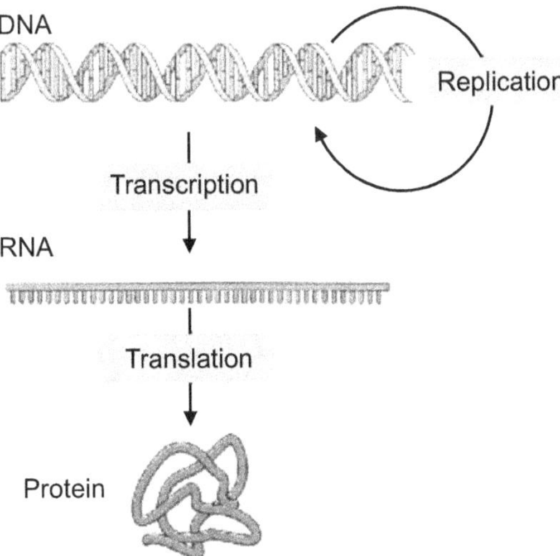

Fig. 8.8: Summary of protein synthesis

QUESTIONS

Short Answer Questions

1. Describe the structure of chromosome.
2. What is deoxyribonucleic acid (DNA).
3. Define translation and transcription process of protein sysntheis.
4. What is gene?
5. Give the functions of chromosomes.

Long Answer Questions

1. Explain the process of protein sysnthesis.

<u>Glossary</u>

<u>**A**</u>

- **Absorption:** Intake of fluids or other substances by cells of the skin or mucous membranes; the passage of digested foods from the gastrointestinal tract into blood or lymph.
- **Acini**: Groups of cells in the pancreas that secrete digestive enzymes.
- **Acrosome:** A lysosome like organelle in the head of a sperm cell containing enzymes that facilitate the penetration of a sperm cell into a secondary oocyte.
- **Action potential:** An electrical signal that propagates along the membrane of a neuron or muscle fiber (cell); a rapid change in membrane potential that involves a depolarization followed by a repolarization.
- **Adenosine triphosphate:** The main energy currency in living cells; used to transfer the chemical energy needed for metabolic reactions.
- **Adrenal glands:** Two glands located superior to each kidney.
- **Aerobic:** Requiring molecular oxygen.
- **Afferent arteriole:** A blood vessel of a kidney that divides into the capillary network called a glomerulus; there is one afferent arteriole for each glomerulus.
- **Aldosterone:** A mineralocorticoid produced by the adrenal cortex that promotes sodium and water reabsorption by the kidneys and potassium excretion in urine.
- **Alpha cell:** A type of cell in the pancreatic islets (islets of Langerhans) in the pancreas that secretes the hormone glucagon.
- **Alveolar macrophage**: Highly phagocytic cell found in the alveolar walls of the lungs.
- **Alveolar sac:** A cluster of alveoli that share a common opening.
- **Alveolus:** A small hollow or cavity; an air sac in the lungs; milk-secreting portion of a mammary gland.
- **Ampulla:** A sac like dilation of a canal or duct.
- **Anabolism:** Synthetic, energy requiring reactions whereby small molecules are built up into larger ones.
- **Anaerobic:** Not requiring oxygen.
- **Androgens:** Masculinizing sex hormones produced by the testes in males and the adrenal cortex in both sexes; responsible for libido (sexual desire); the two main androgens are testosterone and dihydrotestosterone.
- **Anterior pituitary:** Anterior lobe of the pituitary gland. Also called the Adenohypophysis.
- **Anterior root:** The structure composed of axons of motor (efferent) neurons that emerges from the anterior aspect of the spinal cord and extends laterally to join a posterior root, forming a spinal nerve. It is also called as ventral root.
- **Antidiuretic hormone (ADH)**: Hormone produced by neurosecretory cells in the paraventricular and supraoptic nuclei of the hypothalamus that stimulates water

reabsorption from kidney tubule cells into the blood and vasoconstriction of arterioles. It is also called as vasopressin.

- **Antidiuretic:** Substance that inhibits urine formation.
- **Anus:** The distal end and outlet of the rectum.
- **Apocrine gland:** A type of gland in which the secretory products gather at the free end of the secreting cell and are pinched off, along with some of the cytoplasm, to become the secretion, as in mammary glands.
- **Arachnoid mater:** The middle of the three meninges (coverings) of the brain and spinal cord.
- **Arbor vitae:** The white matter tracts of the cerebellum, which have a tree like appearance when seen in mid-sagittal section.
- **Areola:** Any tiny space in a tissue. The pigmented ring around the nipple of the breast.
- **Arytenoid cartilages:** A pair of small, pyramidal cartilages of the larynx that attach to the vocal folds and intrinsic pharyngeal muscles and can move the vocal folds.
- **Ascending colon:** The part of the large intestine that passes superiorly from the cecum to the inferior border of the liver, where it bends at the right colic (hepatic) flexure to become the transverse colon.
- **Ascites:** Abnormal accumulation of serous fluid in the peritoneal cavity.
- **Asthma:** Usually allergic reaction characterized by smooth muscle spasms in bronchi resulting in wheezing and difficult breathing. It is also called bronchial asthma.
- **Astrocyte:** A neuroglial cell having a star shape that participates in brain development and the metabolism of neurotransmitters, helps form the blood–brain barrier, helps maintain the proper balance of K^+ for generation of nerve impulses, and provides a link between neurons and blood vessels.
- **Atrial natriuretic peptide (ANP):** Peptide hormone, produced by the atria of the heart in response to stretching, that inhibits aldosterone production and thus lowers blood pressure; causes natriuresis, increased urinary excretion of sodium.
- **Autonomic ganglion:** A cluster of cell bodies of sympathetic or parasympathetic neurons located outside the central nervous system.
- **Autonomic nervous system (ANS):** Visceral sensory (afferent) and visceral motor (efferent) neurons. Autonomic motor neurons, both sympathetic and parasympathetic, conduct nerve impulses from the central nervous system to smooth muscle, cardiac muscle, and glands. So named because this part of the nervous system was thought to be self-governing or spontaneous.
- **Autosome:** Any chromosome other than the X and Y chromosomes (sex chromosomes).
- **Axon terminal:** Terminal branch of an axon where synaptic vesicles undergo exocytosis to release neurotransmitter molecules.
- **Axon:** The usually single, long process of a nerve cell that propagates a nerve impulse toward the axon terminals.

B

- **Basal ganglia:** Paired clusters of gray matter deep in each cerebral hemisphere including the globus pallidus, putamen, and caudate nucleus.
- **Beta cell:** A type of cell in the pancreatic islets (islets of Langerhans) in the pancreas that secretes the hormone insulin.
- **Beta receptor** A type of adrenergic receptor for epinephrine and norepinephrine; found on visceral effectors innervated by sympathetic postganglionic neurons.
- **Bile:** A secretion of the liver consisting of water, bile salts, bile pigments, cholesterol, lecithin, and several ions; it emulsifies lipids prior to theirdigestion.
- **Bolus:** A soft, rounded mass, usually food, that is swallowed.
- **Brain stem:** The portion of the brain immediately superior to the spinal cord, made up of the medulla oblongata, pons, and midbrain.
- **Brain:** The part of the central nervous system contained within the cranial cavity.
- **Broad ligament:** A double fold of parietal peritoneum attaching the uterus to the side of the pelvic cavity.
- **Broca's area:**Motor area of the brain in the frontal lobe that translates thoughts intospeech. It is also called the motor speech area.
- **Bronchi:** Branches of the respiratory passage way including primary bronchi (the two divisions of the trachea), secondary or lobar bronchi (divisions of the primary bronchi that are distributed to the lobes of the lung), and tertiary or segmental bronchi (divisions of the secondary bronchi).
- **Bronchial tree:** The trachea, bronchi, and their branching structures up to and including the terminal bronchioles.
- **Bronchiole:** Branch of a tertiary bronchus further dividing into terminal bronchioles (distributed to lobules of the lung), which divide into respiratory bronchioles (distributed to alveolar sacs).
- **Bronchitis:** Inflammation of the mucous membrane of the bronchial tree; characterized by hypertrophy and hyperplasia of seromucous glands and goblet cells that line the bronchi which results in a productive cough.
- **Buccal:** Pertaining to the cheek or mouth.
- **Bulb of penis:** Expanded portion of the base of the corpus spongiosum penis.
- **Bulbourethral gland:** One of apair of glands located inferior to the prostate oneither side of the urethra that secretes an alkaline fluid into the cavernous urethra. It is also called as Cowper's gland.

C

- **Calcitonin:**A hormone produced by the parafollicular cells of the thyroid gland that can lower the amount of blood calcium and phosphates by inhibiting bone resorption (breakdown of bone extracellular matrix) and by accelerating uptake of calcium and phosphates into bone matrix.

- **Calyx:** Any cuplike division of the kidney pelvis.
- **Canal:** A narrow tube, channel or passage way.
- **Catabolism:** Chemical reactions that break down complex organic compounds into simple ones, with the net release of energy.
- **Cataract:** Loss of transparency of the lens of the eye or its capsule or both.
- **Cauda equina:** A tail-like array of roots of spinal nerves at the inferior end of the spinal cord.
- **Cecum:** A blind pouch at the proximal end of the large intestine that attaches to the ileum.
- **Central canal:** A microscopic tube running the length of the spinal cord in the gray commissure.
- **Central nervous system:** That portion of the nervous system that consists of the brain and spinal cord.
- **Cerebellar peduncle:** A bundle of nerve axons connecting the cerebellum with the brain stem.
- **Cerebellum:** The part of the brain lying posterior to the medulla oblongata and pons; governs balance and coordinates skilled movements.
- **Cerebral cortex:** The surface of the cerebral hemispheres, 2–4 mm thick, consisting of gray matter; arranged in six layers of neuronal cell bodies in most areas.
- **Cerebral peduncle:** One of a pair of nerve axon bundles located on the anterior surface of the midbrain, conducting nerve impulses between the pons and the cerebral hemispheres.
- **Cerebrospinal fluid:** A fluid produced by ependymal cells that cover choroid plexuses in the ventricles of the brain; the fluid circulates in the ventricles, the central canal, and the subarachnoid space around the brain and spinal cord.
- **Cerebrospinal fluid:** A fluid produced by ependymal cells that cover choroid plexuses in the ventricles of the brain; the fluid circulates in the ventricles, the central canal, and the subarachnoid space around thebrain and spinal cord.
- **Cerebrum:** The two hemispheres of the forebrain (derived from the telencephalon), making up the largest part of the brain.
- **Cervical ganglion:** A cluster of cell bodies of postganglionic sympatheticneurons located in the neck, near the vertebral column.
- **Cervix:** Neck; any constricted portion of an organ, such as the inferior cylindrical part of the uterus.
- **Chief cell:** The secreting cell of a gastric gland that produces pepsinogen, the precursor of the enzyme pepsin, and the enzyme gastric lipase.
- **Cholinergic neuron:** A neuron thatliberates acetylcholine as its neurotransmitter.
- **Choroid:** One of the vascular coats of the eyeball.
- **Chromaffin cell:** Cell that has an affinity for chrome salts, due in part to the presence of the precursors of the neuro transmitter epinephrine; found, among other places, in the adrenal medulla.

- **Chromatid:** One of a pair of identical connected nucleoprotein strands that are joined at the centromere and separate during cell division, each becoming a chromosome of one of the two daughter cells.
- **Chromatin:** The threadlike mass of genetic material, consisting of DNA and histoneproteins, that is present in the nucleus of a non-dividing or interphase cell.
- **Chromosome:** One of the small, thread like structures in the nucleus of a cell, normally 46 in a human diploid cell that bears the genetic material.
- **Chronic obstructive pulmonary disease:** A disease, such as bronchitis or emphysema, in which there is some degree of obstruction of airways and consequent increase in air way resistance.
- **Ciliary body:** One of the three parts of the vascular tunic of the eyeball, the others being the choroid and the iris; includes the ciliary muscle and the ciliary processes.
- **Cilium:** A hair or hair like process projecting from a cell that may be used to move the entire cell or to move substances along the surface of the cell.
- **Clitoris:** An erectile organ of the female, located at the anterior junction of the labia minora, that is homologous to the male penis.
- **Column:** Group of white matter tracts in the spinal cord.
- **Common bile duct:** A tube formed by the union of the common hepatic duct and the cystic duct that empties bile into the duodenum at the hepato pancreatic ampulla.
- **Contraception:** The prevention of fertilization or impregnation without destroying fertility.
- **Corpus albicans:** A white fibrous patch in the ovary that forms after the corpus luteum regresses.
- **Corpus callosum:** The great commissure of the brain between the cerebral hemispheres.
- **Corpus luteum:** A yellowish body in the ovary formed when a follicle has discharged its secondary oocyte; secretes estrogens, progesterone, relaxin, and inhibin.
- **Corpus striatum:** An area in the interior of each cerebral hemisphere composed of the caudate and putamen of the basal ganglia and white matter of the internal capsule, arranged in a striated manner.
- **Cortex**: An outer layer of an organ. The convoluted layer of gray matter covering each cerebral hemisphere.
- **Cranial cavity:** A body cavity formed by the cranial bones and containing the brain.
- **Cranial nerve:** One of 12 pairs of nerves that leave the brain; pass through foramina in the skull; and supply sensory and motor neurons to the head, neck, part of the trunk, and viscera of the thorax and abdomen. Each is designated by a Roman numeral and a name.
- **Craniosacral outflow:** The axons of parasympathetic preganglionic neurons, which have their cell bodies located in nuclei in the brain stem and in the lateral gray matter of the sacral portion of the spinal cord.

- **Cranium:** The skeleton of the skull that protects the brain and the organs of sight, hearing, and balance; includes the frontal, parietal, temporal, occipital, sphenoid, and ethmoid bones.
- **Cystic duct**: The duct that carries bile from the gall bladder to the common bile duct.
- **Cystitis:** Inflammation of the urinary bladder.

D

- **Deciduous:** Falling off or being shed seasonally or at a particular stage of development.
- **Defecation:** The discharge of faeces from the rectum.
- **Deglutition:** The act of swallowing.
- **Dehydration:** Excessive loss of water from the body or its parts.
- **Delta cell:** A cell in the pancreatic islets (islets of Langerhans) in the pancreas that secretes somatostatin.
- **Dendrite:** A neuronal process that carries electrical signals, usually graded potentials, toward the cell body.
- **Dental caries:** Gradual demineralization of the enamel and dentin of a tooth that may invade the pulp and alveolar bone.
- **Dentin:** The bony tissues of a tooth enclosing the pulp cavity.
- **Deoxyribonucleic acid:** A nucleic acid constructed of nucleotides consisting of one of four bases (adenine, cytosine, guanine, or thymine), deoxyribose, and a phosphate group; encoded in the nucleotides is genetic information.
- **Descending colon:** The part of the large intestine descending from the left colic (splenic) flexure to the level of the left iliac crest.
- **Detrusor muscle:** Smooth muscle that forms the wall of the urinary bladder.
- **Diaphragm:** Any partition that separates one area from another, especially the dome shaped skeletal muscle between the thoracic and abdominal cavities.
- **Diencephalon:** A part of the brain consisting of the thalamus, hypothalamus, and epithalamus.
- **Digestion:** The mechanical and chemical breakdown of food to simple molecules that can be absorbed and used by body cells.
- **Diploid:** Having the number of chromosomes characteristically found in the somatic cells of an organism; having two haploid sets of chromosomes, one each from the mother and father.
- **Diuretic:** A chemical that increases urine volume by decreasing reabsorption of water, usually by inhibiting sodium reabsorption.
- **Ductus (vas) deferens:** The duct that carries sperm from the epididymis to the ejaculatory duct.
- **Ductus epididymis:** A tightly coiled tube inside the epididymis, distinguished into a head, body, and tail, in which sperm undergo maturation.
- **Duodenum:** The first 25 cm part of the small intestine, which connects the stomach and the ileum.

- **Dura mater:** The outermost of the three meninges (coverings) of the brain and spinal cord.
- **Dysmenorrhea:** Painful menstruation.
- **Dyspnoea:** Shortness of breath; painful breathing.

E

- **Effector:** An organ of the body, either a muscle or a gland that is innervated by somatic or autonomic motor neurons.
- **Efferent arteriole:** A vessel of the renal vascular system that carries blood from a glomerulus to a peritubular capillary.
- **Efferent ducts:** A series of coiled tubes that transport sperm from the rete testis to the epididymis.
- **Ejaculation:** The reflex ejection or expulsion of semen from the penis.
- **Ejaculatory duct:** A tube that transports sperm from the ductus (vas) deferens to the prostatic urethra.
- **Emphysema:** A lung disorder in which alveolar walls disintegrate, producing abnormally large air spaces and loss of elasticity in the lungs; typically caused by exposure to cigarette smoke.
- **Enamel:** The hard, white substance covering the crown of a tooth.
- **Endocrine gland:** A gland that secretes hormones into interstitial fluid and then the blood; a ductless gland.
- **Endocrinology:** The science concerned with the structure and functions of endocrine glands and the diagnosis and treatment of disorders of the endocrine system.
- **Endometrium:** The mucous membrane lining the uterus.
- **Enteroendocrine cell:** A cell of the mucosa of the gastrointestinal tract that secretes a hormone that governs function of the GI tract; hormones secreted include gastrin, cholecystokinin, glucose-dependent insulino tropic peptide (GIP), and secretin.
- **Epididymis:** A comma-shaped organ that lies along the posterior border of the testis and contains the ductus epididymis, in which sperm undergo maturation.
- **Epiglottis:** A large, leaf-shaped piece of cartilage lying on top of the larynx, attached to the thyroid cartilage; its unattached portion is free to move up and down to cover the glottis during swallowing.
- **Epinephrine:** Hormone secreted by the adrenal medulla that produces actions similar to those that result from sympathetic stimulation.
- **Epithalamus:** Part of the diencephalon superior and posterior to the thalamus, comprising the pineal gland and associated structures.
- **Esophagus:** The hollow muscular tube that connects the pharynx and the stomach.
- **Estrogens:** Feminizing sex hormones produced by the ovaries; govern development of oocytes, maintenance of female reproductive structures, and appearance of secondary sex characteristics; also affect fluid and electrolyte balance, and protein anabolism. Examples are β estradiol, estrone, and estriol.

- **Excretion:** The process of eliminating waste products from the body; also the products excreted.
- **Exhalation:** Breathing out; expelling air from the lungs into the atmosphere. Also called expiration.
- **Exocrine gland:** A gland that secretes its products into ducts that carry the secretions into body cavities, into the lumen of an organ, or to the outer surface of the body.
- **External nares:** The openings into the nasal cavity on the exterior of the body.
- **External respiration:** The exchange of respiratory gases between the lungs and blood. Also called **pulmonary respiration.**

F

- **F cell:** A cell in the pancreatic islets (islets of Langerhans) that secretes pancreatic polypeptide.
- **Falciform ligament:** A sheet of parietal peritoneum between the two principal lobes of the liver.
- **Falx cerebelli:** A small triangular process of the dura mater attached to the occipital bone in the posterior cranial fossa and projecting inward between the two cerebellar hemispheres.
- **Falx cerebri:** A fold of the dura mater extending deep into the longitudinal fissure between the two cerebral hemispheres.
- **Feces:** Material discharged from the rectum and made up of bacteria, excretions, and food residue. Also called stool.
- **Female reproductive cycle:** General term for the ovarian and uterine cycles, the hormonal changes that accompany them, and cyclic changes in the breasts and cervix; includes changes in the endometrium of a non pregnant female that prepares the lining of the uterus to receive a fertilized ovum.
- **Fertilization**: Penetration of a secondary oocyte by a sperm cell, meiotic division of secondary oocyte to form an ovum, and subsequent union of the nuclei of the gametes.
- **Filiform papilla:** One of the conical projections that are distributed in parallel rows over the anterior two-thirds of the tongue and lack taste buds.
- **Filtration:** The flow of a liquid through a filter (or membrane that acts like a filter) due to a hydrostatic pressure; occurs in capillaries due to blood pressure.
- **Fimbriae:** Finger like structures, especially the lateral ends of the uterine (Fallopian) tubes.
- **Follicle:** A small secretory sac or cavity; the group of cells that contains a developing oocyte in the ovaries.
- **Follicle-stimulating hormone:** Hormone secreted by the anterior pituitary; it initiates development of ova and stimulates the ovaries to secrete estrogens in females, and initiates sperm production in males.

- **Fourth ventricle:** A cavity filled with cerebrospinal fluid within the brain lying between the cerebellum and the medulla oblongata and pons.
- **Frontal plane:** A plane at a right angle to a Mid-sagittal plane that divides the body or organs into anterior and posterior portions.
- **Fundus:** The part of a hollow organ farthest from the opening.
- **Fungiform papilla:** A mushroom like elevation on the upper surface of the tongue appearing as a red dot; most contain taste buds.

G

- **Gallbladder:** A small pouch, located inferior to the liver, that stores bile and empties by means of the cystic duct.
- **Gamete:** A male or female reproductive cell; a sperm cell or secondary oocyte.
- **Ganglion:** Usually, a group of neuronal cell bodies lying outside the central nervous system.
- **Gastric glands:** Glands in the mucosa of the stomach composed of cells that empty their secretions into narrow channels called gastric pits.
- **Gastroenterology:** The medical specialty that deals with the structure, function, diagnosis, and treatment of diseases of the stomach and intestines.
- **Gastrointestinal tract:** A continuous tube running through the ventral body cavity extending from the mouth to the anus. It is also called the alimentary canal.
- **Gene:** Biological unit of heredity; a segmentof DNA located in a definite position on a particular chromosome; a sequence of DNA that codesfor a particular mRNA, rRNA, or tRNA.
- **Genetics** The study of genes and heredity.
- **Gingivae:** Gums. They cover the alveolar processes of the mandible and maxilla and extend slightly into each socket.
- **Gland:** Specialized epithelial cell or cells that secrete substances; may be exocrine or endocrine.
- **Glans penis:** The slightly enlarged region at the distal end of the penis.
- **Glaucoma:** An eye disorder in which there is increased intraocular pressure due to an excess of aqueous humor.
- **Glomerular capsule:** A double walled globe at the proximal end of a nephron that encloses the glomerular capillaries.
- **Glomerular filtrate:** The fluid produced when blood is filtered by the filtration membrane in the glomeruli of the kidneys.
- **Glomerular filtration:** The first step in urine formationin which substances in blood pass through the filtration membrane and the filtrate enters the proximal convoluted tubule of a nephron.
- **Glomerulus:** A rounded mass of nerves or blood vessels, especially the microscopic tuft of capillaries that is surrounded by the glomerular (Bowman's) capsule of each kidney tubule.

- **Glucagon:** A hormone produced by the alpha cells of the pancreatic islets (islets of Langerhans) that increases blood glucose level.
- **Glucocorticoids:** Hormones secreted by the cortex of the adrenal gland, especially cortisol that influence glucose metabolism.
- **Glucose:** A hexose (six-carbon sugar), $C_6H_{12}O_6$, that is a major energy source for theproduction of ATP by body cells.
- **Glucosuria:** The presence of glucose in the urine; may be temporary or pathological. Also called **glycosuria.**
- **Glycogen:** A highly branched polymer of glucose containing thousands of subunits; functions as a compact store of glucose molecules in liver and muscle fibers (cells).
- **Goblet cell:** A goblet-shaped unicellular gland that secretes mucus; present in epithelium of the airways and intestines.
- **Goiter**: An enlarged thyroid gland.
- **Gonad:** A gland that produces gametes and hormones; the ovary in the female and the testis in the male.
- **Gonadotropic hormone:** Anterior pituitary hormone that affects the gonads.
- **Gray matter:** Areas in the central nervous system and ganglia containing neuronal cell bodies, dendrites, unmyelinated axons, axon terminals and neuroglia.

H

- **Haploid cell:** Having half the number of chromosomes characteristically found in the somatic cells of an organism; characteristic of mature gametes.
- **Hard palate:** The anterior portion of the roof of the mouth, formed by the maxillae and palatine bones and lined by mucous membrane.
- **Hepatic duct:** A duct that receives bile from the bile capillaries. Small hepatic ducts merge to form the larger right and left hepatic ducts that unite to leave the liver as the common hepatic duct.
- **Hepatocyte:** A liver cell.
- **Hilum:** An area, depression, or pit where blood vessels and nerves enter or leave an organ.
- **Hormone:** A secretion of endocrine cells that alters the physiological activity of target cells of the body.
- **Horn** An area of gray matter (anterior, lateral, or posterior) in the spinal cord.
- **Human chorionic gonadotropin:** A hormone produced bythe developing placenta that maintains the corpus luteum.
- **Human growth hormone:** Hormone secreted by the anterior pituitary that stimulates growth of body tissues, especially skeletal and muscular tissues.
- **Hymen:** A thin fold of vascularized mucous membrane at the vaginal orifice.
- **Hypothalamus:** A portion of the diencephalon, lying beneath the thalamus and forming the floor and part of the wall of the third ventricle.

I

- **Ileocecal sphincter:** A fold of mucous membrane that guards the opening from the ileum into the large intestine
- **Ileum:** The terminal part of the small intestine.
- **Infundibulum**: The stalk like structure that attaches the pituitary gland to the hypothalamus of the brain. The funnel-shaped, open, distal end of the uterine (Fallopian) tube.
- **Ingestion:** The taking in of food, liquids, or drugs, by mouth.
- **Inhalation:**The act of drawing air into the lungs.
- **Inheritance** The acquisition of body traits by transmission of genetic information from parents to offspring.
- **Inhibin** A hormone secreted by the gonads that inhibits release of follicle-stimulating hormone(FSH) by the anterior pituitary.
- **Inhibiting hormone:** Hormone secreted by the hypothalamus that can suppress secretion of hormones by the anterior pituitary.
- **Insulin:** A hormone produced by the beta cells of a pancreatic islet (islet of Langerhans) that decreases the blood glucose level.
- **Internal nares:** The two openings posterior to the nasal cavities opening into the nasopharynx.
- **Internal respiration:** The exchange of respiratory gases between blood and body cells. It is also called tissue respiration.
- **Isthmus:** A narrow strip of tissue or narrow passage connecting two larger parts.

J

- **Jejunum:** The middle part of the small intestine.
- **Juxtaglomerular apparatus:** Consists of the macula densa (cells of the distal convoluted tubule adjacent to the afferent and efferent arteriole) and juxtaglomerular cells; secretes renin when blood pressure starts to fall.

K

- **Keratin:** An insoluble protein found in the hair, nails, and other keratinized tissues of the epidermis.
- **Keratinocyte:** The most numerous of the epidermal cells; produces keratin.
- **Kidney:** One of the paired reddish organs located in the lumbar region that regulates the composition, volume, and pressure of blood and produces urine.

L

- **Labia majora:** Two longitudinal folds of skin extending downward and backward from the mons pubis of the female.
- **Labia minora:** Two small folds of mucous membrane lying medial to the labia majora of the female.
- **Labor:** The process of giving birth in which a fetus is expelled from the uterus through the vagina.
- **Lactation:** The secretion and ejection of milk by the mammary glands.
- **Langerhans cell:** Epidermal dendritic cell that functions as an antigen-presenting cell (APC) during an immune response.
- **Large intestine:** The portion of the gastro intestinal tract extending from the ileum of the small intestine to the anus, divided structurally into the cecum, colon, rectum, and anal canal.
- **Laryngopharynx:** The inferior portion of the pharynx, extending downward from the level of the hyoid bone that divides posteriorly into the esophagus and anteriorly into the larynx.
- **Larynx:** The voice box, a short passage way that connects the pharynx with the trachea.
- **Lateral:** Farther from the midline of the body or a structure.
- **Leydig cell:** A type of cell that secretes testosterone; located in the connective tissue between seminiferous tubules in a mature testis.
- **Limbic system:** A part of the forebrain, sometimes termed the visceral brain, concerned with various aspects of emotion and behaviour; includes the limbic lobe, dentate gyrus, amygdala, septal nuclei, mammillary bodies, anterior thalamic nucleus, olfactory bulbs, and bundles of myelinated axons.
- **Liver:** Large organ under the diaphragm that occupiesmost of the right hypochondriac region and part of the epigastric region.
- **Lungs:** Main organs of respiration that lie on eitherside of the heart in the thoracic cavity.
- **Luteinizing hormone:** Ahormone secreted by the anterior pituitary that stimulates ovulation, stimulates progesterone secretion by the corpus luteum, and readies the mammary glands for milk secretion in females; stimulates testosterone secretion by the testes in males.

M

- **Mammary gland:** Modified sudoriferous (sweat) gland of the female that produces milk for the nourishment of the young.
- **Mature follicle:** A large, fluid-filled follicle containing a secondary oocyte and surrounding granulosa cells that secrete estrogens.
- **Medulla oblongata:** The most inferior part of the brain stem.
- **Medulla:** An inner layer of an organ, such as the medulla of the kidneys.
- **Medullary rhythmicity area:** The neurons of the respiratory center in the medulla oblongata that control the basic rhythm of respiration.

- **Melanocyte:** A pigmented cell, located between or beneath cells of the deepest layer of the epidermis, that synthesizes melanin.
- **Melanocyte-stimulating hormone:** A hormone secreted by the anterior pituitary that stimulates the dispersion of melanin granules in melanocytes in amphibians; continued administration produces darkening of skin in humans.
- **Melatonin:** A hormone secreted by the pineal gland that helps set the timing of the body's biological clock
- **Meninges:** Three membranes covering the brain and spinal cord, called the dura mater, arachnoid mater, and pia mater.
- **Menstrual cycle:** A series of changes in the endometrium of a non pregnant female that prepares the lining of the uterus to receive a fertilized ovum.
- **Menstruation:** Periodic discharge of blood, tissue fluid, mucus, and epithelial cells that usually lasts for 5 days; caused by a sudden reduction in estrogens and progesterone.
- **Metabolism:** All the biochemical reactions that occur within an organism, including the synthetic (anabolic) reactions and decomposition (catabolic) reactions.
- **Microglia:** Neuroglial cells that carry on phagocytosis.
- **Microvilli:** Microscopic, finger like projections of the plasma membranes of cells that increase surface area for absorption, especially in the small intestine and proximal convoluted tubules of the kidneys.
- **Micturition:** The act of expelling urine from the urinary bladder.
- **Midbrain:** The part of the brain between the pons and the diencephalon.
- **Mineralocorticoids:** A group of hormones of the adrenal cortex that help regulate sodium and potassium balance.
- **Mons pubis:** The rounded, fatty prominence over the pubic symphysis, covered by coarse pubic hair.
- **Mucous cell:** A unicellular gland that secretes mucus. Two types are mucous neck cells and surface mucous cells in the stomach.
- **Mucous membrane:** A membrane that lines a body cavity that opens to the exterior.
- **Mucus:** The thick fluid secretion of goblet cells, mucous cells, mucous glands, and mucous membranes.
- **Muscular tissue:** A tissue specialized to produce motion in response to muscle action potentials by its qualities of contractility, extensibility, elasticity, and excitability; types include skeletal, cardiac, and smooth.
- **Muscularis:** A muscular layer (coat or tunic) of an organ.
- **Myometrium**: The smooth muscle layer of the uterus.

N

- **Nasal cavity:** A mucosa-lined cavity on either side of the nasal septum that opens on to the face at the external nares and into the Nasopharynx at the internal nares.
- **Nasal septum:** A vertical partition composed of bone (perpendicular plate of ethmoid and vomer) and cartilage, covered with a mucous membrane, separating the nasal cavity into left and right sides.

- **Nasopharynx:** The superior portion of the pharynx, lying posterior to the nose and extending inferiorly to the soft palate.
- **Nephron:** The functional unit of the kidney.
- **Nerve** A cordlike bundle of neuronal axons and/or dendrites and associated connective tissue coursing together outside the central nervous system.
- **Nerve fiber:** Any process (axon or dendrite) projecting from the cell body of a neuron.
- **Nerve impulse:** A wave of depolarization and repolarization that self-propagates along the plasma membrane of a neuron.
- **Nervous tissue:** Tissue containing neurons that initiate and conduct nerve impulses to coordinate homeostasis, and neuroglia that provide support and nourishment to neurons.
- **Neuroglia:** Cells of the nervous system that perform various supportive functions. The neuroglias of the central nervous system are the astrocytes, oligodendrocytes, microglia, and ependymal cells; neuroglia of the peripheral nervous system includes Schwann cells and satellite cells.
- **Neurolemma:** The peripheral, nucleated cytoplasmic layer of the Schwann cell.
- **Neurology:** The study of the normal functioning and disorders of the nervous system.
- **Neuromuscular junction:** A synapse between the axon terminals of a motor neuron and the sarcolemma of a muscle fiber (cell).
- **Neuron:** A nerve cell, consisting of a cell body, dendrites, and an axon.
- **Neurotransmitter:** One of a variety of molecules within axon terminals that are released into the synaptic cleft in response to a nerve impulse and that change the membrane potential of the post synaptic neuron.
- **Nipple:** A pigmented, wrinkled projection on the surface of the breast that is the location of the openings of the lactiferous ducts for milk release.
- **Norepinephrine:** A hormone secreted by the adrenal medulla that produces actions similar to those that result from sympathetic stimulation.

O

- **Oligodendrocyte:** A neuroglial cell that supports neurons and produces amyelin sheath around axons of neurons of the central nervous system.
- **Oliguria:** Daily urinary output usually less than 250 ml.
- **Oogenesis:** Formation and development of female gametes (oocytes).
- **Organogenesis:** The formation of body organs and systems.
- **Oropharynx:** The intermediate portion of the pharynx, lying posterior to themouth and extending from the soft palate to the hyoid bone.
- **Osmoreceptor:** Receptor in the hypothalamus that is sensitive to changes in blood osmolarity and, in response to high osmolarity (low water concentration), stimulates synthesis and release of antidiuretic hormone (ADH).
- **Ovarian follicle:** A general name for oocytes (immature ova) in any stage of development, along with their surrounding epithelial cells.

- **Ovarian ligament:** A rounded cord of connective tissue that attaches the ovary to the uterus.
- **Ovary:** Female gonad that produces oocytes and the estrogens, progesterone, inhibin, and relaxin hormones
- **Ovulation:** The rupture of a mature ovarian (Graafian) follicle with discharge of a secondary oocyte into the pelvic cavity.
- **Ovum:** The female reproductive or germ cell; an egg cell; arises through completion of meiosisin a secondary oocyte after penetration by a sperm.
- **Oxytocin:** A hormone secreted by neurosecretory cells in the paraventricular and supraoptic nuclei of the hypothalamus that stimulates contraction of smooth muscle in the pregnant uterus and myoepithelial cells around the ducts of mammary glands.

P

- **Palate:** The horizontal structure separating the oral and the nasal cavities; the roof of the mouth.
- **Pancreas:** A soft, oblong organ lying along the greater curvature of the stomach and connected by a duct to the duodenum.
- **Pancreatic duct:** A single large tube that unites with the common bile duct from the liver and gall bladder and drains pancreatic juice into the duodenum at the hepatopancreatic ampulla.
- **Pancreatic islet:** A cluster of endocrine gland cells in the pancreas that secretes insulin, glucagon, somatostatin, and pancreatic polypeptide.
- **Papilla:** A small nipple-shaped projection or elevation.
- **Parasympathetic division:** One of the two subdivisions of the autonomic nervous system, having cell bodies of preganglionic neurons in nuclei in the brain stem and in the lateral gray horn of the sacral portion of the spinal cord; primarily concerned with activities that conserve and restore body energy.
- **Parathyroid gland:** One of usually four small endocrine glands embedded in the posterior surfaces of the lateral lobes of the thyroid gland.
- **Parathyroid hormone:** A hormone secreted by the chief (principal) cells of the parathyroid glands that increases blood calcium level and decreases blood phosphate level.
- **Parietal cell:** A type of secretory cell in gastric glands that produces hydrochloric acid and intrinsic factor.
- **Parietal pleura:** The outer layer of the serous pleural membrane that encloses and protects the lungs; the layer that is attached to the wall of the pleural cavity.
- **Parkinson disease:** Progressive degeneration of the basal ganglia and substantia nigra of the cerebrum resulting in decreased production of dopamine (DA) that leads to tremor, slowing of voluntary movements, and muscle weakness.
- **Parotid gland:** One of the paired salivary glands located inferior and anterior to the ears and connected to the oral cavity via. a duct that opens into the inside of the cheek opposite the maxillary (upper) second molar tooth.

- **Pars intermedia:** A small avascular zone between the anterior and posterior pituitary glands.
- **Parturition:** Act of giving birth to young; childbirth, delivery
- **Pelvis:** The basin like structure formed by the two hip bones, the sacrum, and the coccyx. The expanded, proximal portion of the ureter, lying within the kidney and into which the major calyces open.
- **Penis:** The organ of urination and copulation in males; used to deposit semen into the female vagina.
- **Pepsin:** Protein-digesting enzyme secreted by chief cells of the stomach in the inactive form pepsinogen, which is converted to active pepsin by hydrochloric acid.
- **Peptic ulcer:** An ulcer that develops in areas of the gastrointestinal tract exposed to hydrochloric acid; classified as a gastric ulcer if in the lesser curvature of the stomach and as a duodenal ulcer if in the first part of the duodenum.
- **Perimetrium:** The serosa of the uterus.
- **Periodontal disease:** A collective term for conditions characterized by degeneration of gingivae, alveolar bone, periodontal ligament, and cementum.
- **Peripheral nervous system:** The part of the nervous system that lies outside the central nervous system, consisting of nerves and ganglia.
- **Peristalsis:** Successive muscular contractions along the wall of a hollow muscular structure.
- **pH:** A measure of the concentration of hydrogen ions (H^+) in a solution. The pH scale extends from 0 to 14, with a value of 7 expressing neutrality, values lower than 7 expressing increasing acidity, and values higher than 7 expressing increasing alkalinity.
- **Pharynx:** The throat; a tube that starts at the internal nares and runs partway down the neck, where it opens into the esophagus posteriorly and the larynx anteriorly.
- **Pia mater:** The innermost of the three meninges (coverings) of the brain and spinal cord.
- **Pituitary gland:** A small endocrine gland occupying the hypophyseal fossa of the sphenoid bone and attached to the hypothalamus by the infundibulum.
- **Placenta:** The special structure through which the exchange of materials between fetal and maternal circulations occurs.
- **Polyuria:** An excessive production of urine.
- **Pons:** The part of the brain stem that forms a "bridge" between the medulla oblongata and the midbrain, anterior to the cerebellum.
- **Postcentral gyrus:** Gyrus of cerebral cortex located immediately posterior to the central sulcus; contains the primary somato sensory area.
- **Posterior pituitary:** Posterior lobe of the pituitary gland.
- **Posterior root ganglion:** A group of cell bodies of sensory neurons and their supporting cells located along the posterior root of aspinal nerve. It is also called a dorsal (sensory) root ganglion.

- **Posterior root:** The structure composed of sensoryaxons lying between a spinal nerve and the dorsolateral aspect of the spinal cord. It also called the dorsal (sensory) root.
- **Postganglionic neuron:** The second autonomic motor neuron in anautonomic pathway, having its cell body and dendriteslocated in an autonomic ganglion and its unmyelinated axon ending at cardiac muscle,smooth muscle, or a gland.
- **Postsynaptic neuron:** The nervecell that is activated by the release of a neurotransmitter from another neuron and carries nerve impulses away from the synapse.
- **Precentral gyrus:** Gyrus of cerebral cortex located immediately anterior to the central sulcus; contains the primary motor area.
- **Preganglionic neuron:** The first autonomic motor neuron in an autonomic pathway, with its cell body and dendrites in the brain or spinal cord and its myelinated axon ending at an autonomic ganglion, where it synapses with a postganglionic neuron.
- **Pregnancy:** Sequence of events that normally includes fertilization, implantation, embryonic growth, and fetal growth and terminates in birth.
- **Primary motor area:** A region of the cerebral cortexin the precentral gyrus of the frontal lobe of the cerebrum that controls specific muscles orgroups of muscles.
- **Primary somatosensory area:** A region of the cerebral cortex posterior to the central sulcus in the postcentral gyrus of the parietal lobe of the cerebrum that localizes exactly the points of the body where somatic sensations originate.
- **Progesterone:** A female sex hormone produced by the ovaries that helps prepare the endometrium of the uterus for implantation of a fertilized ovum and the mammary glands for milk secretion.
- **Prolactin:** A hormone secreted by the anterior pituitary that initiates and maintains milk secretion by the mammary glands.
- **Proliferation:** Rapid and repeated reproduction of new parts, especially cells.
- **Prostate:** A doughnut-shaped gland inferior to the urinary bladder that surrounds the superior portion of the male urethra and secretes a slightly acidic solution that contributes to sperm motility and viability.
- **Pyloric sphincter:** A thickened ring of smooth muscle through which the pylorus of the stomach communicates with the duodenum. It is also called the pyloric valve.
- **Pyramid** (PIR-a-mid) A pointed or cone-shaped structure. One of two roughly triangular structures on the anterior aspect of the medulla oblongata composed of the largest motor tracts that run from the cerebral cortex to the spinal cord. A triangular structure in the renal medulla.

R

- **Receptor:** A specialized cell or a distal portion of a neuron that responds to a specific sensory modality, such as touch, pressure, cold, light, or sound, and converts it to an electrical signal.

- **Rectum:** The last 20 cm (8 in.) of the gastrointestinal tract, from the sigmoid colon to the anus.
- **Reflex arc:** The most basic conduction pathway through the nervous system, connecting a receptor and an effector and consisting of a receptor, a sensory neuron, an integrating center in the central nervous system, a motor neuron, and an effector.
- **Relaxin:** A female hormone produced by the ovaries and placenta that increases flexibility of the pubic symphysis and helps dilate the uterine cervix to ease delivery of a baby.
- **Renal corpuscle:** A glomerular (Bowman's) capsule and its enclosed glomerulus.
- **Renal pelvis:** A cavity in the center of the kidney formed by the expanded, proximal portion of the ureter, lying within the kidney, and into which the major calyces open.
- **Renal pyramid:** A triangular structure in the renal medulla containing the straight segments of renal tubules and the vasa recta.
- **Renal:** Pertaining to the kidneys.
- **Reproduction:** The formation of new cells for growth, repair, or replacement; the production of a new individual.
- **Respiration:** Overall exchange of gases between the atmosphere, blood, and body cells consisting of pulmonary ventilation, external respiration, and internal respiration.
- **Respiratory center:** Neurons in the pons and medulla oblongata of the brain stem that regulate the rate and depth of pulmonary ventilation.
- **Root canal:** A narrow extension of the pulp cavity lying within the root of a tooth.
- **Root of penis:** Attached portion of penis that consists of the bulb and crura.

<u>S</u>

- **Saliva:** A clear, alkaline, somewhat viscous secretion produced mostly by the three pairs of salivary glands; contains various salts, mucin, lysozyme, salivary amylase, and lingual lipase (produced by glands in the tongue).
- **Salivary amylase:** An enzyme in saliva that initiates the chemical breakdown of starch.
- **Salivary gland:** One of three pairs of glands that lieexternal to the mouth and pour their secretory product (saliva) into ducts that empty into the oral cavity; the parotid, submandibular, and sublingual glands.
- **Scrotum:** A skin-covered pouch that contains the testes and their accessory structures
- **Semen:** A fluid discharged at ejaculation by a male that consists of a mixture of sperm and the secretions of the seminiferous tubules, seminal vesicles, prostate, and bulbo urethral (Cowper's) glands.
- **Seminal vesicle:** One of a pair of convoluted, pouch like structures, lying posterior and inferior to the urinary bladder and anterior to the rectum, that secrete a component of semen into the ejaculatory ducts.

- **Seminiferous tubule:** A tightly coiled duct, located in the testis, where sperm are produced.
- **Sensory area:** A region of the cerebral cortex concerned with the interpretation of sensory impulses.
- **Sensory neurons:** Neurons that carry sensory information from cranial and spinal nerves into the brain and spinal cord or from a lower to a higher level in the spinal cord and brain.
- **Sertoli cell:** A supporting cell in the seminiferous tubules that secretes fluid for supplying nutrients to sperm and the hormone inhibin, removes excess cytoplasm from Spermatogenic cells, and mediates the effects of FSH and testosterone on spermatogenesis.
- **Sigmoid colon:** The S-shaped part of the large intestine that begins at the level of the left iliac crest, projects medially, and terminates at the rectum at about the level of the third sacral vertebra.
- **Small intestine:** A long tube of the gastrointestinal tract that begins at the pyloric sphincter of the stomach, coils through the central and inferior part of the abdominal cavity, and ends at the large intestine; divided into three segments: duodenum, jejunum, and ileum.
- **Soft palate:** The posterior portion of the roof of the mouth, extending from the palatine bones to the uvula. It is a muscular partition lined with mucous membrane.
- **Somatic nervous system:** The portion of the peripheral nervous system consisting of somatic sensory (afferent) neurons and somatic motor (efferent) neurons.
- **Sperm cell:** A mature male gamete.
- **Spermatic cord:** A supporting structure of the male reproductive system, extending from a testis to the deep inguinal ring, that includes the ductus (vas) deferens, arteries, veins, lymphatic vessels, nerves, cremaster muscle, and connective tissue.
- **Spermatogenesis:** The formation and development of sperm in the seminiferous tubules of the testes.
- **Spermiogenesis:** The maturation of spermatids into sperm.
- **Sphincter:** A circular muscle that constricts an opening.
- **Spinal cord:** A mass of nerve tissue located in the vertebral canal from which 31 pairs of spinal nerves originate.
- **Stomach** The J-shaped enlargement of the gastrointestinal tract directly inferior to the diaphragm in the epigastric, umbilical, and left hypochondriac regions of the abdomen, between the esophagus and small intestine.
- **Stratum basalis:** The layer of the endometrium next to the myometrium that is maintained during menstruation and gestation and produces a new stratum functionalis following menstruation or parturition.
- **Stratum functionalis:** The layer of the endometrium next to the uterine cavity that is shed during menstruation and that forms the maternal portion of the placenta during gestation.

- **Stretch receptor:** Receptor in the walls of blood vessels, airways, or organs that monitors the amount of stretching.
- **Subarachnoid space:** A space between the arachnoid mater and the pia mater that surrounds the brain and spinal cord and through which cerebrospinal fluid circulates.
- **Subdural space:** A space between the dura mater and the arachnoid mater of the brain and spinal cord that contains a small amount of fluid.
- **Sublingual gland:** One of a pair of salivary glands situated in the floor of the mouth deep to the mucous membrane and to the side of the lingual frenulum, with a duct that opens into the floor of the mouth.
- **Submandibular gland:** One of a pair of salivary glands found inferior to the base of the tongue deep to the mucous membrane in the posterior part of the floor of the mouth, posterior to the sublingual glands, with a duct situated to the side of the lingual frenulum.
- **Submucosa:** A layer of connective tissue located deep to a mucous membrane, as inthe gastrointestinal tract or the urinary bladder; the submucosa connects the mucosa to the muscularis layer.
- **Sulcus:** A groove or depression between parts, especially between the convolutions of the brain.
- **Sympathetic trunk ganglion:** A cluster of cell bodies of sympathetic post ganglionic neurons lateral to the vertebral column, close to the body of a vertebra.
- **Synaptic end bulb:** Expanded distal end of an axon terminal that contains synaptic vesicles.
- **Synaptic vesicle:** Membrane-enclosed sac in asynaptic end bulb that stores neurotransmitters.

T

- **Tentorium cerebelli:** A transverse shelf of dura mater that forms a partition between the occipital lobe of the cerebral hemispheres and the cerebellum and that covers the cerebellum.
- **Testis:** Male gonad that produces sperm and the hormones testosterone and inhibin.
- **Testosterone:** A male sex hormone (androgen) secreted by interstitial endocrinocytes (Leydig cells) of a mature testis; needed for development of sperm; together with a second androgen termed dihydrotestosterone, controls the growth and development of male reproductive organs, secondary sex characteristics, and body growth.
- **Thalamus:** A large, oval structure located bilaterally on either side of the third ventricle, consisting of two masses of gray matter organized into nuclei; main relay center for sensory impulses ascending to the cerebral cortex.
- **Thalamus:** A large, oval structure located bilaterally on either side of the third ventricle, consisting of two masses of gray matter organized into nuclei; main relay center for sensory impulses ascending to the cerebral cortex.

- **Third ventricle:** A slit like cavity between the right and left halves of the thalamus and between the lateral ventricles of the brain.
- **Thoracic cavity:** Cavity superior to the diaphragm that contains two pleural cavities, the mediastinum, and the pericardial cavity.
- **Thoracolumbar outflow:** The axons of sympathetic preganglionic neurons, which have their cell bodies in the lateral gray columns of the thoracic segments and first two or three lumbar segments of the spinal cord.
- **Thyroid cartilage:** The largest single cartilage of the larynx, consisting of two fused plates that form the anterior wall of the larynx.
- **Thyroid follicle:** Spherical sac that forms the parenchyma of the thyroid gland and consists of follicular cells that produce thyroxine (T_4) and triiodothyronine (T_3).
- **Thyroid gland:** An endocrine gland with right and left lateral lobes on either side of the trachea connected by an isthmus; located anterior to the trachea just inferior to the cricoid cartilage; secretes thyroxine (T_4), triiodothyronine (T_3), and calcitonin.
- **Thyroid-stimulating hormone:** A hormone secreted by the anterior pituitary that stimulates the synthesis and secretion of thyroxine (T_4) and triiodothyronine (T_3).
- **Thyroxine:** A hormone secreted by the thyroid gland that regulates metabolism, growth and development, and the activity of the nervous system.
- **Tongue:** A large skeletal muscle covered by a mucous membrane located on the floor of the oral cavity.
- **Trachea:** Tubular air passage way extending from the larynx to the fifth thoracic vertebra.
- **Transverse colon:** The portion of the large intestine extending across the abdomen from the right colic (hepatic) flexure to the left colic (splenic) flexure.
- **Tubular reabsorption:** The movement of filtrate from renal tubules back into blood in response to the body's specific needs.
- **Tubular secretion:** The movement of substances in blood into renal tubular fluid in response to the body's specific needs.
- **Tunica albuginea:** Adense white fibrous capsule covering a testis or deep to the surface of an ovary.
- **Tunica externa:** The superficial coat of an artery or vein, composed mostly of elastic and collagen fibers.

U

- **Ureter:** One of two tubes that connect the kidney with the urinary bladder.
- **Urethra:** The duct from the urinary bladder to the exterior of the body that conveys urine in females and urine and semen in males.
- **Urinalysis:** An analysis of the volume and physical, chemical, and microscopic properties of urine.
- **Urinary bladder:** A hollow, muscular organ situated in the pelvic cavity posterior to the pubic symphysis; receives urine via two ureters and stores urine until it is excreted through the urethra.

- **Urine:** The fluid produced by the kidneys that contains wastes and excess materials; excreted from the body through the urethra.
- **Uterine tube:** Duct that transports ova from the ovary to the uterus.
- **Uterus:** The hollow, muscular organ in females that is the site of menstruation, implantation, development of the fetus, and labor.

V

- **Vagina:** A muscular, tubular organ that leads from the uterus to the vestibule, situated between the urinary bladder and the rectum of the female.
- **Vallate papilla:** One of the circular projections that is arranged in an inverted V shaped row at the back of the tongue; the largest of the elevations on the upper surface of the tongue containing taste buds.
- **Vas:** A vessel or duct.
- **Vermis:** The central constricted area of the cerebellum that separates the two cerebellar hemispheres.
- **Vertebral column:** The 26 vertebrae of an adult and 33 vertebrae of a child; encloses and protects the spinal cord and serves as a point of attachment for the ribs and back muscles.
- **Vocal cords:** Pair of mucous membrane folds below the ventricular folds that function in voice production.
- **Vulva:** Collective designation for the external genitalia of the female.

W

- **White matter:** Aggregations or bundles of myelinated and unmyelinated axons located in the brain and spinal cord.

Z

- **Zona fasciculata:** The middle zone of the adrenal cortex consisting of cellsarranged in long, straight cords that secrete glucocorticoidhormones, mainly cortisol.
- **Zona glomerulosa:** The outer zone of the adrenal cortex, directly under the connective tissue covering, consisting of cells arranged in arched loops or round balls that secrete mineralocorticoid hormones, mainly aldosterone.
- **Zona pellucida:** Clear glycoprotein layer between a secondary oocyte and the surrounding granulosa cells of the corona radiata.
- **Zona reticularis:** The inner zone of the adrenal cortex, consisting of cords of branching cells that secrete sex hormones, chiefly androgens.
- **Zygote:** The single cell resulting from the union of male and female gametes; the fertilized ovum.

✼✼✼

Index

****

Bibliography

- **Agarwal PK,** Anatomy Physiology and Pathophysiology-III, Pragati Prakashan, First Edition, 2009.
- **Agur AR and Dalley AF,** Grants Atlas of anatomy, Lippincott Williams and Wilkins, Eleventh Edition, 2005.
- **Applegate E,** The Anatomy and Physiology Learning System, Saunders Elsevier, Third Edition, 2006.
- **Bhise, Yadav and Burkul**, Anatomy Physiology and Health Education, Nirali Prakashan, Second Edition, 2003.
- **Chakraborty N and Chakraborty D,** Fundamentals of Human Anatomy, Volume-III, New Central Book Agency, First Edition Reprint, 2004.
- **Chatterjee CC,** Human Physiology. Medical Allied Agency, Volume-I, Eleventh Edition Reprint, 2005.
- **Chaudhuri SK,** Concise Medical Physiology, New Central Book Agency, Sixth Edition, 2008.
- **Chaurasia BD,** Human Anatomy, Volume-I, CBS Publishers and Distributors, Third Edition Reprint, 2004.
- **Dandiya, Zafer and Zafer**, Health Education and community Pharmacy, Vallabh Prakashan, First Edition Reprint 2003.
- **Goyal RK and Patel NM,** Practical Anatomy Physiology and Biochemistry, Shah Prakashan, Eleventh Edition, 2008. Edition
- **Goyal RK,** Basics of Human Anatomy and Physiology, BS Prakashan, Second Edition, 2006.
- **Gupta AK**, Handbook of Health Education and Community Pharmacy, CBS Publishers and Distributers Private Ltd., First Edition Reprint 2012.
- **Guyton AC and Hall JE,** Textbook of Medical Physiology, Saunders Elsevier, First Edition Reprint, 2011.
- **Moore KL and Dalley AF,** Clinically Oriented Anatomy, Lippincott Williams and Wilkins, Third Edition, 1992.
- **Moore KL, Dalley AF and Agur AR,** Clinically Oriented Anatomy, Lippincott Williams and Wilkins, Sixth Edition, 2009.
- **Pal GK and Pal P,** Textbook of Practical Physiology, Universities Press, First Edition, 2011.
- **Pathak NK,** Easy Book of Anatomy, New Central Book Agency, First Edition, 2008.
- **Phate RP,** Anatomy, Physiology and Health Education, Career Publication, Second Edition, 2003.
- **Satyanarayana U**, Biochemistry, Books and Allied Private Ltd, Second Revised Edition, 2002.
- **Seeley RR, Stephens TD and Tate P,** Essentials of Anatomy and Physiology, Mc Graw Hill, Fourth Edition, 2002.
- **Thibodeau GA and Patton KT,** Anthony's Textbook of Anatomy and Physiology, Elsevier, Seventeenth Edition, 1999.
- **Tortora GJ and Grabowski SR,** Principles of Anatomy and Physiology, John Wiley and Sons, Inc. Tenth Edition, 2005.
- **Waugh A and Grant A,** Anatomy and Physiology in Health and Illness, Churchill Livingstone, Eleventh Edition, 2010.
- **Williams PL,** Grays Anatomy, Churchill Livingstone, Thirty Eighth Editions, 2000.

***